DIPLOMA IN INTERNAL

Hypertension after Menopause

Hypertension after Menopause

Edited by

M. Stimpel · A. Zanchetti

Walter de Gruyter
Berlin · New York 1997

Editors

M. Stimpel, M. D.
Assistant Professor of Medicine
Medical School
University of Cologne
D-50931 Cologne
Germany

Mail address:
Frieding Straße 13
D-40625 Düsseldorf
Germany

A. Zanchetti, M. D.
Professor of Medicine
Centro di Fisiologia
Clinica e Ipertensione
Policlinico
I-20122 Milano
Italy

The editors wish to acknowledge the excellent editorial assistance of Dr. Brigitte Koch and Dagmar I. Prüsse.

Die Deutsche Bibliothek – Cataloging-in-Publication-Data

Hypertension after menopause / ed. by M. Stimpel ; A. Zanchetti. –
Berlin ; New York : de Gruyter, 1997
ISBN 3-11-015518-4
NE: Stimpel, Michael [Hrsg.]

Printed in Germany

Typesetting: Arthur Collignon GmbH, Berlin. – Printing: Gerike GmbH, Berlin. – Binding: Mikolai, Berlin. – Cover design: Rudolf Hübler, Berlin

Contributors

Bieniaszewski, Leszek, M. D., Ph.D.
Hypertension and Cardiovascular Rehabilitation Unit, Department of Molecular and Cardiovascular Research, University of Leuven, Belgium and Department of Hypertension and Diabetology, Medical Academy of Gdansk, Gdansk, Poland

Brosens, Ivo, M. D., Ph.D.
Gynecology and Obstetrics Unit, Department of Developmental Biology, University of Leuven, B-3000 Leuven, Belgium

Carugo, Stefano, M. D.
Cattedra Medicina Interna, Universita di Milano and Ospedale San Gerardo, I-20052 Monza, Milano, Italy

Chambers, Timothy, J., Ph.D., M. D.
Professor of Histopathology, Department of Histopathology, St. George's Hospital, Cranmer Terrace, Tooting, London SW17 ORE, United Kingdom

Chen, Yiu-Fai, Ph.D.
Professor of Medicine, The University of Alabama at Birmingham, 1034 Zeigler Research Buildung, 703 South 19th Street, Birmingham, Alabama 35294–0007, USA

Courivaux, Jean-Michel
Centre Hospitalier F. H. Manhès, 8 Grande Rue, Fleury-Mérogis, F-91712 Ste-Geneviève-des-Bois Cedex, France

Fagard, Robert, M. D., Ph.D.
Hypertension and Cardiovascular Rehabilitation Unit, Department of Molecular and Cardiovascular Research, University of Leuven, B-3000 Leuven, Belgium

Failla, Monica, M. D.
Cattedra Medicina Interna, Universita di Milano and Ospedale San Gerardo, I-20052 Monza, Milano, Italy

Giannattasio, Cristina, M. D.
Assistant Professor of Medicine, Cattedra Medicina Interna, Universita di Milano and Ospedale San Gerardo, I-20052 Monza, Milano, Italy

Godsland, Ian, Ph.D.
Senior Lecturer, Wynn Division of Metabolic Medicine, Imperial College School of Medicine at the National Heart and Lung Institute, 21 Wellington Road, London NW8 9SQ, United Kingdom

Hatton, Ruth, BSc
Department of Histopathology, St. George's Hospital, Cranmer Terrace, Tooting, London SW17 ORE, United Kingdom

Jee, Webster, S. S., Ph.D.
Professor, Radiobiology Division, University of Utah, Salt Lake City, Utah, UT 84112 USA

Koch, Brigitte, Ph.D.
Schwarz Pharma AG, Department of Clinical Research, D-40789 Monheim, Germany

London, Gerard, M. D.
Centre Hospitalier F. H. Manhès, 8 Grande Rue, Fleury-Mérogis, F-91712 Ste-Geneviève-des-Bois Cedex, France

Mancia, Giuseppe, M. D.
Professor of Medicine, Cattedra Medicina Interna, Universita di Milano and Ospedale San Gerardo, I-20052 Monza, Milano; Centro Auxologico Italiano, Milano, Italy

Mangoni, Arduino A., M. D.
Cattedra Medicina Interna, Universita di Milano and Ospedale San Gerardo, I-20052 Monza, Milano, Italy.

Neyses, Ludwig, M. D.
Assistant Professor of Medicine, Department of Medicine, University of Würzburg, Josef-Schneider-Strasse 2, D-97080 Würzburg, Germany

Oparil, Suzanne, M. D.
Professor of Medicine, The University of Alabama at Birmingham, 1034 Zeigler Research Buildung, 703 South 19th Street, Birmingham, AL 35294–0007, USA

Pelzer, Theo, M. D.
Department of Medicine, University of Würzburg, Josef-Schneider-Strasse 2, D-97080 Würzburg, Germany

Safar, Michel, M. D.
Professor of Medicine, Service de Médicine Interne, Hôpital Broussais, 96 Rue Didot, F-75014 Paris, France

Staessen, Jan, A., M. D., Ph.D.
Hypertension and Cardiovascular Rehabilitation Unit, Department of Molecular and Cardiovascular Research, University of Leuven, B-3000 Leuven, Belgium

Stella, Maria Luisa, M. D.
Cattedra Medicina Interna and Centro di Fisiologia Clinica Universita di Milano Ospedale Maggiore and Ospedale San Gerardo, I-20052 Monza, Milano, Italy

Stevenson, John C., MB, FRCP
Director, Wynn Divison of Metabolic Medicine, Imperial College School of Medicine at the National Heart and Lung Institute, 21 Wellington Road, London NW8 9SQ, United Kingdom

Stimpel, Michael, M. D.
Assistant Professor of Medicine, Medical School, University of Cologne, D-50931 Cologne, and Schwarz Pharma AG, Department of Clinical Research, D-40789 Monheim, Germany

Weber, Michael, A., M. D.
Professor of Medicine, Department of Medicine, The Brookdale University Hospital and Medical Center, Brooklyn, NY 11212−3198, USA

Zanchetti, Alberto, M. D.
Professor of Medicine, Centro di Fisiologia, Clinica e Ipertensione, Policlinico, I-20122 Milano, Italy

Contents

1 Introduction

Michael Stimpel and Alberto Zanchetti

This international Workshop on "Hypertension in Postmenopausal Women" the proceedings of which are published in this volume, was the second in a series which began in Monte Carlo two years ago (1). There is no doubt that the topic of this meeting is one which deserves increased scientific attention. Cardiovascular disease in women has long been disregarded as being of minor importance, and hypertension likewise is often considered to be a low risk condition in women. In times when much emphasis is put on the cost-effectiveness of treatment and the evaluation of the absolute rather than the relative risk and benefit of disease and treatment respectively, there is a rising possibility of women being denied the benefit of antihypertensive therapy on the basis of a broad and superficial assumption that cardiovascular risk in women is low. In fact, only recently has scientific attention been drawn to dividing line, represented by the menopausal period, after which age-related blood pressure changes are greater in women than in men, hypertension becomes more prevalent in females, and global cardiovascular risk in women reaches a comparable level as in men. Concomitant diseases such as type 2 diabetes mellitus also become highly prevalent in females. We must understand better the causes and mechanisms of these menopause-related changes: Is the age-dependent increase in cardiovascular disease simply greater in women? Are all changes related to hormonal loss? How much is the increased risk due to metabolic changes or to vascular and cardiac functional and structural changes? These and many other questions need to be answered before we can provide a coherent preventive and therapeutic strategy towards cardiovascular disease in postmenopausal women.

Well-known experts addressed several of these questions at this meeting. It is, however, not without signifance that, at a meeting primarily concerned with hypertension and the menopause, attention has also been paid to another menopause-related condition, osteoporosis. Indeed, there is mounting evidence that local vascular factors may play a significant role in the occurrence of osteoporosis, with the implication of the endothelium and the ubiquitous generation of angiotensin II.

While these new areas of research continue to develop, we must also address the problem as to how we can best treat the postmenopausal hypertensive patient. The new interest in this question is displayed in the development of a new ACE-inhibitor, moexipril. A number of the efficacy and safety studies have been carried out exclusively in postmenopausal hypertensive patients with and without hormone replacement therapy, and we are finally beginning to obtain valuable information on how to approach therapy in these patients.

Reference

1. Safar, M, Stimpel M, Zanchetti A (eds). Hypertension in postmenopausal women. Springer-Verlag 1994, Berlin Heidelberg.

2 Cardiovascular disease in women: an overview

Suzanne Oparil and Yiu-Fai Chen

Introduction

Epidemiological and clinical studies have defined a sexually dimorphic pattern in the development of atherosclerotic vascular disease in humans (1). The incidence of cardiovascular disease is low in premenopausal women, but rises steadily after the menopause, although never attaining levels of age-matched men (2). Age-adjusted rates of fatal and nonfatal myocardial infarction are higher in men than in women in all age groups, but the gap narrows in later decades. Cardiovascular disease is the leading cause of death in women in the U. S., accounting for almost 500,000 deaths per year (Figure 2.1) (3). Half of all cardiovascular deaths are due to heart attack, and 40 percent of heart attacks in women are fatal. Heart attack kills more than 5 times as many women in the U. S. as breast cancer, and stroke, the third cause of death and leading cause of disability, kills twice as many women as breast cancer (Figure 2.2) (3). Disability due to cardiovascular disease is also a major problem for women: 36 percent of women in the age range 55–64 with ischemic heart disease are disabled; 55 percent of women over age 75 that are so afflicted are disabled (4). In the United States in 1996, the estimated cost of cardiovascular disease in medical expenses and lost productivity will be $151 billion (U. S. dollars) (3). Well over half of these health care costs are related to disease in women.

Postmenopausal women on estrogen replacement therapy have less severe coronary artery disease and a lower risk of cardiovascular mortality than women without hormone treatment (5). Thus, estrogens inhibit the development of atherosclerotic cardiovascular disease in women (6). The mechanisms of this vasoprotective effect are complex and involve alterations in lipid metabolism, endothelial function, smooth muscle cell proliferation and associated extracellular matrix formation, and vascular reactivity. Evidence that other sex hormones, including androgens and progestins, can also alter these processes, is emerging. This chapter will review the problem of cardiovascular disease in women, with emphasis on the effects of the sex hormones, particularly estrogen, on the vasculature. The effects of postmenopausal hormone replacement on cardiovascular risk will be reviewed specifically.

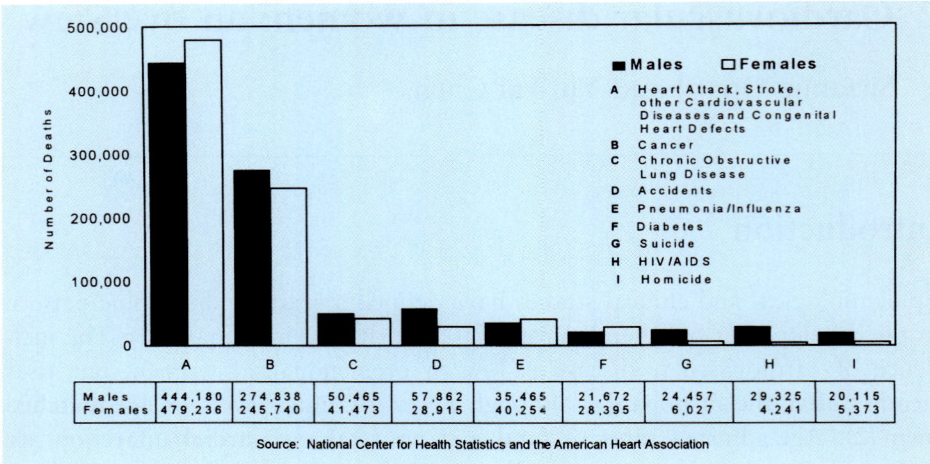

Figure 2.1: Leading causes of death in the USA in 1992 (adapted from reference 3, with permission).

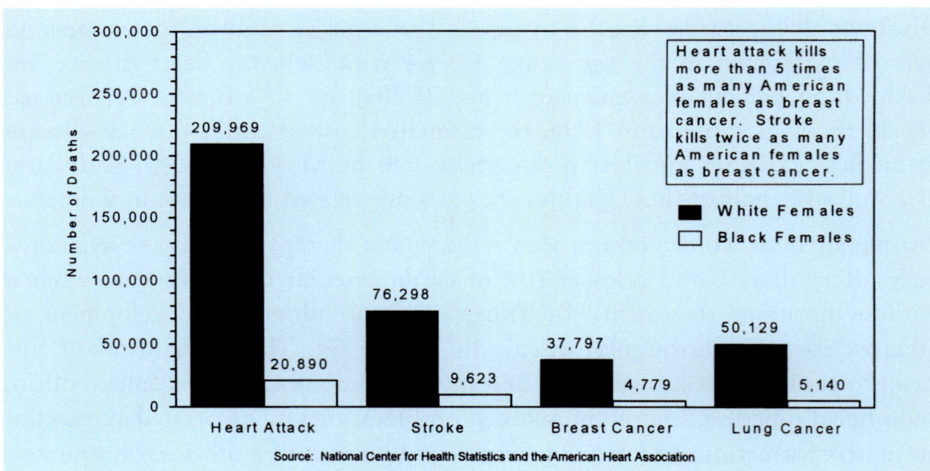

Figure 2.2: Heart attack and stoke vs. breast and lung cancer deaths in while and black females in the USA in 1992 (reproduced from reference 3, with permission).

Cardiovascular risk factors and preventive strategies in women

Smoking

Cigarette smoking produces a dose-related increase in cardiovascular risk in women as well as men (Figure 2.3). This increased risk is reversible with smoking cessation, reaching the level of risk of nonsmokers within 3–5 years regardless of the amount smoked, duration of smoking, or age at cessation (7–9). The rate of smoking cessation is currently lower among women than among men, and more vigorous efforts to discourage smoking among women are needed.

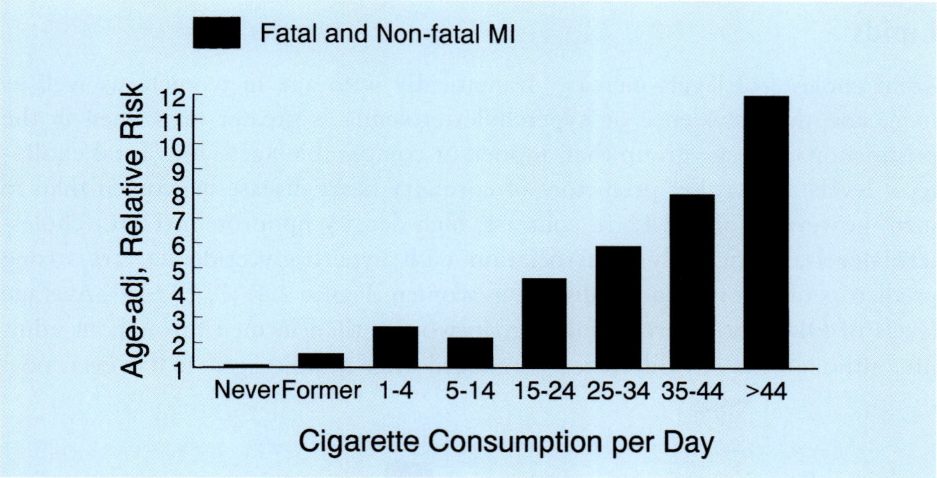

Figure 2.3: Smoking and CHD (coronary heart disease) risk in women. Source: Nurses' Health Study – 6 year follow-up (adapted from reference 8, with permission).

Hypertension

Systolic blood pressure and the prevalence of hypertension, particularly, systolic hypertension, increase dramatically with age in women (10). Hypertension is significantly less common in women than in men before the time of the menopause; thereafter its prevalence in women increases, reaching levels significantly higher than those in men of the same age. Whether the menopause per se contributes to the age-related increase in blood pressure in women is controversial. Cross-sectional studies have found higher blood pressures among post-menopausal than premenopausal women at a given age (11, 12), while longitudinal studies have not shown a significant rise in blood pressure at the time of menopause (13–15). New data, using men as controls, indicate that the menopause, per se, is related to accelerated blood pressure increases and that there is an increased prevalence of hypertension in a carefully studied population (see Staessen J, Chapter 3). At present it is uncertain whether the menopause-related increase in blood pressure is related to estrogen withdrawal, overproduction of pituitary hormones, weight gain, and/or a combination of these factors and other, yet undefined neurohumoral influences. This is an increasingly important clinical problem in the aging population because of the extremely high prevalence – up to 80% – of hypertension in elderly women and because elevated blood pressure, especially systolic blood pressure, is such an important risk factor for acute coronary events and cardiovascular mortality in women.

Lipids

Total cholesterol levels increase dramatically with age in women, as well as men, and the prevalence of hypercholesterolemia is greater in women in the postmenopausal age group than in men at comparable ages (16). Total cholesterol levels are weaker predictors of coronary heart disease in women than in men, however (Table 2.1). In contrast, high density lipoprotein (HDL) cholesterol levels, particularly in association with hypertriglyceridemia, are strong predictors of coronary heart disease in women (Figure 2.4) (7, 17–19). Average levels of HDL cholesterol are higher in women than in men throughout adult life, although the sex difference is reduced after middle age. It has been pos-

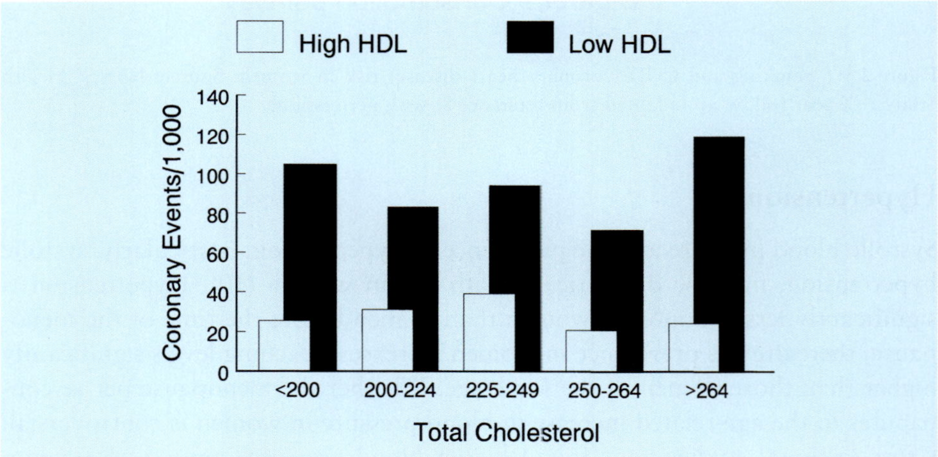

Figure 2.4: Incidence of definite coronary events in women over 20 years of follow-up by age, total serum cholesterol and HDL cholesterol. Drawn with data from reference 18 with permission.

tulated that HDL cholesterol may partly account for the sex difference in coronary heart disease risk, particularly since HDL appears to be more protective in women than in men (20, 21).

Table 2.1: Relative risk (RR) of coronary heart disease by sex. Epidemiologic follow-up study of NHANES I.

Risk Factor	Men RR (95% CI)	Women RR (95% CI)
Hypertension	1.5 (1.3, 1.7)	1.5 (1.3, 1.8)
High cholesterol	1.4 (1.2, 1.6)	1.1 (0.9, 1.2)
Diabetes	1.9 (1.5, 2.5)	2.4 (1.9, 3.0)
Overweight	1.3 (1.1, 1.5)	1.4 (1.2, 1.6)
Smoking	1.6 (1.4, 1.8)	1.8 (1.5, 2.1)

Source: MMWR 1992; 41: 528. (n = 12, 402; mean F/U 12.4y; RR controlled for other variables).

Diabetes mellitus

Diabetes is a more important risk factor for coronary heart disease in women than in men, negating the protective effect of female gender (Table 2.1, Figure 2.5) (19, 22). The Nurses' Health Study showed that maturity onset diabetes was associated with a 3–7-fold increase in risk of a cardiovascular event (23). After 45 years of age, women are twice as likely as men to develop diabetes mellitus (24). Fourteen year follow-up data from the Rancho Bernardo Study

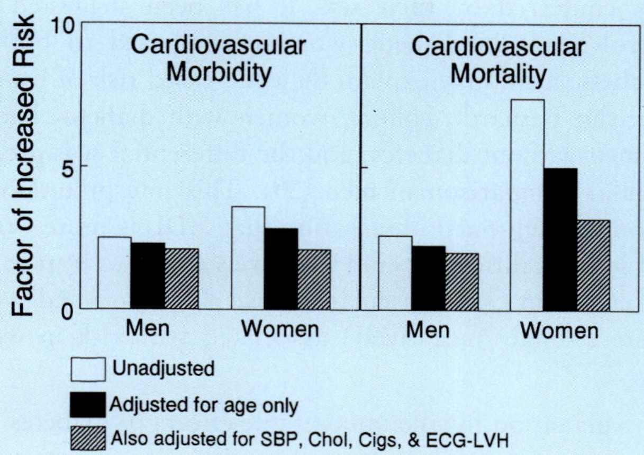

Figure 2.5: Relative risk of cardiovascular events in diabetic vs. nondiabetic men and women ages 45 to 74 years: Framingham Study, 20-year follow-up. Reproduced from reference 38 with permission.

examined the sex-specific effect of non-insulin dependent diabetes mellitus on the risk of ischemic heart disease in a geographically defined population of men and women aged 40–79 years (22). There was a strong positive relationship between fasting plasma glucose levels and coronary heart disease mortality in women. Further, the relative hazard of ischemic heart disease death in diabetics vs nondiabetics was 1.8 in men and 3.3 in women, after adjusting for age, and 1.9 and 3.3 respectively, after adjusting for age, systolic blood pressure, cholesterol, body mass index, and cigarette smoking using the Cox regression model. Thus, diabetes imposes a greater risk of heart disease in women than in men, and the sex difference is independent of other cardiovascular risk factors (22, 25–27), although both men and women with diabetes tend to be more hyperlipidemic, more hypertensive and more obese than nondiabetics. The sex difference in the independent contribution of diabetes to fatal heart disease in the Rancho Bernardo Study was largely explained by the persistently more favorable survival rate of women (than men) without diabetes. The female survival advantage among nondiabetics persisted throughout the 14 year follow-up period, while survival in diabetic women declined to, but not below, the level observed for men after 11 years. Thus, the diabetes-by-sex interaction was not due to higher rates in female vs. male diabetics, but rather to the lower rates in female vs. male nondiabetics (22).

The mechanisms by which diabetes accelerates the natural history of vascular disease are poorly understood, and likely do not relate to hyperglycemia per se. There are clear interactions with other modifiable risk factors, such as hypertension, lipid abnormalities, and obesity, but these factors do not fully explain why diabetic women lose the protective effect against cardiovascular disease usually conferred by their sex. It has been suggested that reduced HDL cholesterol levels in diabetic women, compared to both nondiabetic women and diabetic men, may explain their increased risk of heart disease (22, 28). In the Rancho Bernardo cohort, women with diabetes had lower HDL levels than women without diabetes, and the differential was greater than that found in a similar comparison in men (29). This interpretation is consistent with the previously mentioned observation that HDL is more cardioprotective in women than in men: differences in HDL levels could, at least in part, account for the sex difference in cardiovascular disease risk associated with diabetes if HDL were more strongly (negatively) associated with risk in women than in men.

An additional explanation for the unfavorable effects of diabetes on cardiovascular disease in women is increased insulin resistance with attendant increases in central (male pattern) obesity and androgenicity (22). Women with non-insulin dependent diabetes mellitus typically have insulin resistance, hyperinsulinemia and central obesity, and this constellation of findings is associated with increased androgenicity (30,31). Central obesity in women is strongly inversely correlated with HDL_2 cholesterol levels: HDL_2 is even more strongly correlated with central obesity than with sex (32). The mechanisms of the interactions between androgens and insulin metabolism are poorly understood, although a number of hypotheses have been put forth (33, 34). These interactions, whatever their mechanisms are, likely contribute importantly to sex differences in heart disease risk in both diabetics and non-diabetics (22).

Fibrinogen

Data from Framingham indicate that there is a significant positive relationship between plasma fibrinogen levels and coronary heart disease risk in both sexes (35). Fibrinogen levels increase with age in both sexes and are higher in women than in men at all ages. Observational studies and limited clinical trial data suggest that fibrinogen levels are significantly lower in women taking postmenopausal hormone replacement therapy than in untreated postmenopausal women (36, 37). The magnitude of this effect would be sufficient to double the risk of heart disease, according to Framingham data (35). Mechanisms that have been adduced to explain the enhanced cardiovascular risk associated with increased fibrinogen levels include increased blood viscosity, hypercoagulability, increased platelet aggregation and altered distensibility of erythrocytes. It has also been suggested that circulating fibrinogen levels may reflect the extent of atherosclerotic vascular damage in a subject since high concentrations of fibrinogen have been found in developing lesions and an association has been noted between fibrin accumulation and binding of LDL to plaque. The increased tendency to thrombosis in subjects with elevated fibrinogen levels may predispose to vascular occlusion at the site of advancing atheromata, predisposing to acute clinical events.

Menopause and hormone replacement therapy

The incidence of coronary heart disease in women increases dramatically in middle age. Data from Framingham indicate that there is a 12-fold increase in the incidence of heart attack in women from age 35–44, when most are still menstruating, to age 55–64, when most are postmenopausal (Figure 2.6) (38). Whether this is related to the menopause or to other factors, such as age, weight gain, and cigarette smoking, is controversial (7, 13, 39). When controlled for age and smoking status, most observational studies indicate that natural menopause is not associated with an abrupt increase in coronary risk. In contrast, surgical menopause (bilateral oophorectomy) is associated with a 2–2 fold increase in coronary heart disease risk (39). Estrogen replacement therapy appears to eliminate this increase in risk.

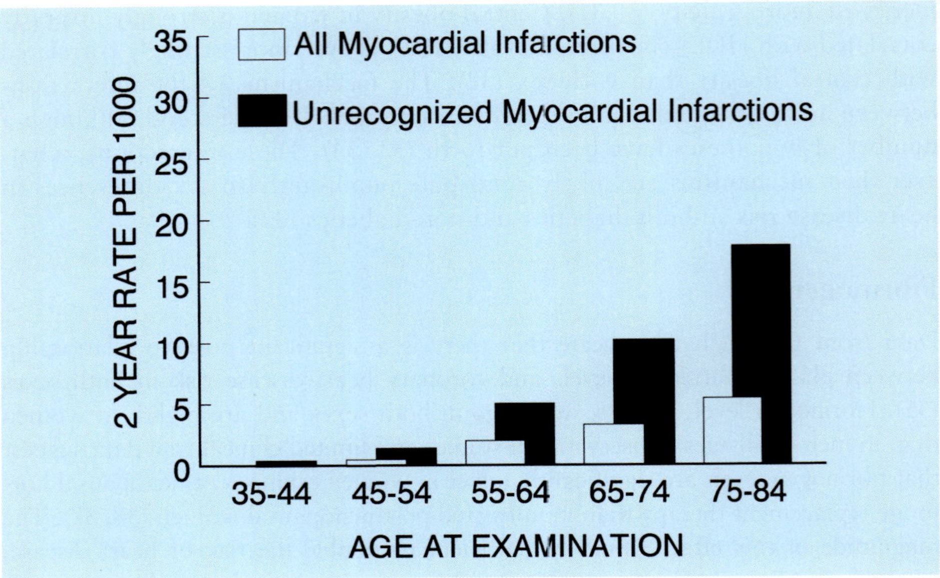

Figure 2.6: Incidence of myocardial infarction by age in women: 26-year follow-up, Framingham Study. Reproduced from reference 38 with permission.

Meta-analyses of observational studies suggest a 50% reduction in heart disease risk in postmenopausal women taking estrogen replacement therapy (40). However, such studies have the severe limitation of treatment selection bias: women who are taking postmenopausal hormone replacement therapy tend to be healthier, better educated, more attentive to lifestyle modification strategies for reducing cardiovascular risk and to have better health care (41). Accordingly, prospective, randomized trials are being carried out to assess the impact of postmenopausal hormone replacement therapy on cardiovascular risk factors and event rates.

The Postmenopausal Estrogen/Progestin Interventions (PEPI) Trial is a prospective, randomized, double-blind, placebo-controlled trial sponsored by the U. S. National Institutes of Health that is assessing differences among placebo, unopposed estrogen, and each of three estrogen/progestin regimens on selected heart disease risk factors in healthy postmenopausal women (42). Primary end points are systolic blood pressure, HDL cholesterol, serum insulin, and fibrinogen. At 3 years of follow-up, estrogen alone and in combination with progestin increased HDL and lowered low-density lipoprotein (LDL) cholesterol and fibrinogen levels (Figure 2.7). Unopposed estrogen was the optimal regimen for reducing cardiovascular disease risk, but was associated with high rates of endometrial hyperplasia and hysterectomy (34% and 6%, respectively). In women with an uterus, conjugated equine estrogen combined with micronized progesterone had the most favorable effect on HDL cholesterol with no excess risk of endometrial hyperplasia. The PEPI trial did not test oral estradiol or any transdermal estrogen preparation. Whether transdermal estrogen shares the positive effect on the lipid profile that has been described for oral conjugated estrogen (43–46) is a matter of debate. Recent data suggest that transdermal estrogen has positive effects on lipids in postmenopausal women (see Stevenson JC, chapter 4). Further study using recently developed preparations and delivery systems for transdermal estrogen is needed to resolve this issue.

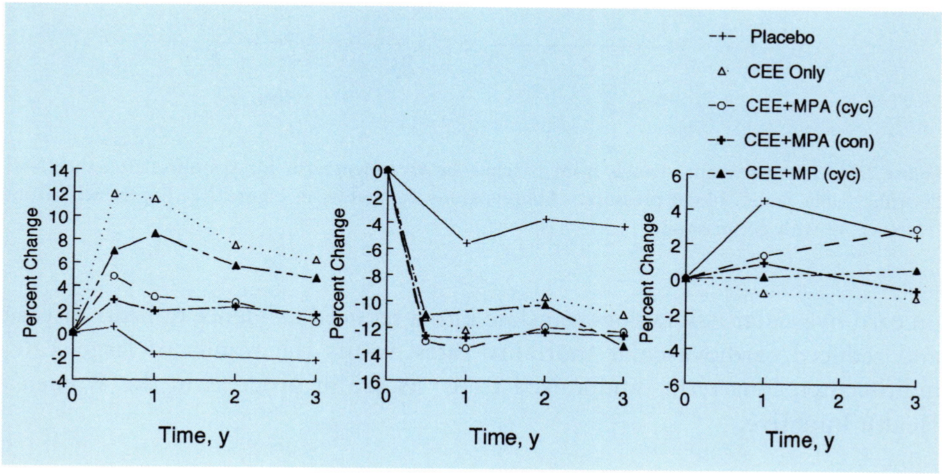

Figure 2.7: Mean percent change from baseline by treatment arm for HDL cholesterol (left panel), LDL cholesterol (middle panel) and fibrinogen (right panel). CEE = conjugated equine estrogen; MPA = medroxy progesterone acetate; CYC = cyclic administration (days 1–12 of each month); con = administered daily; MP = micronized progesterone. Reproduced from reference 42 with permission.

In the PEPI trial, systolic blood pressure increased in parallel with weight gain in all treatment groups; diastolic blood pressure remained close to baseline levels (Figure 2.8). The absence of a treatment effect on blood pressure in these normotensive subjects is consistent with previous reports that hormone replacement therapy does not alter blood pressure in postmenopausal women with hypertension (36, 47, 48).

Taken together, the results of the PEPI trial provide strong evidence that estrogen alone or combined with progestin has a cardioprotective effect in postmenopausal women, particularly those with preexisting coronary disease or at high risk for developing coronary disease (40, 42). Whether these beneficial effects

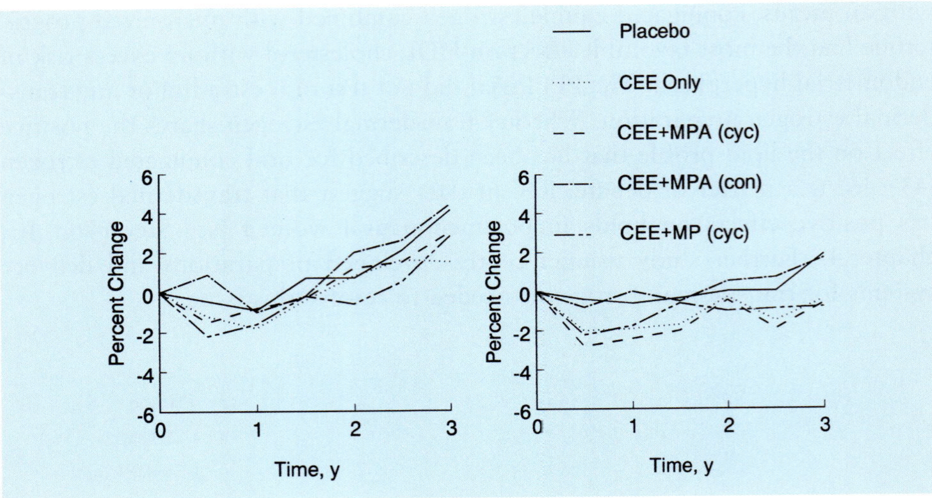

Figure 2.8: Mean percent change from baseline by treatment arm for systolic (left panel) and diastolic (right panel) blood pressure. Abbreviations defined as in Figure 2.7. Reproduced from reference 42 with permission.

on cardiovascular risk factors translate into a reduced incidence of heart disease and reduced cardiovascular mortality rates awaits the results of large-scale, multi-center, long-term randomized trials, as are in progress in the Women's Health Initiative.

Mechanisms of estrogen-induced vasoprotection

The cardioprotection afforded by postmenopausal estrogen replacement therapy is mediated by five major effects: altered lipid metabolism; enhanced endothelial cell function; inhibition of smooth muscle cell migration and proliferation following vascular injury; inhibition of extracellular matrix formation, and enhanced vasodilator responses to stimuli of nitric oxide (NO) synthesis and release. Approximately 30% of the antiatherosclerotic effects of estrogens in humans have been attributed to alterations in plasma lipid and lipoprotein levels, principally elevations in HDL cholesterol, HDL_2, and apoliproprotein A-I (2, 49). Retardation in arterial lesion development can occur in response to estrogen treatment in the absence of alterations in serum cholesterol levels, indicating that other effects can account for some of the vasoprotection afforded by these compounds (50). Many of these direct vasoprotective effects are mediated by the endothelium. These include enhancement of endothelial degradation of LDL cholesterol, antioxidant actions on LDL particles in macrophages, suppression of collagen and elastin synthesis, and restoration of endothelium-dependent vasodilator mechanisms post injury (51–56). Further, estrogen inhibits Ca^{2+} influx through voltage-dependent Ca^{2+} channels in vascular smooth muscle cells (VSMCs), reducing vasoconstrictor responses to a variety of pressors, and causes direct hyperpolarization of resting VSMCs (57). Estrogen also stimulates prostacyclin biosynthesis in cultured VSMCs (58).

The endothelium plays a central role in the control of vascular tone and the growth of the blood vessel wall, mainly through synthesis and release of endothelium-derived relaxing factor (EDRF), which has been shown to be NO (59). NO is both a vasorelaxant and an antimitogen for VSMCs. Release of NO in response to infused acetylcholine, the standard test for assessing endothelium-dependent vascular tone, is responsive to both acute and chronic estrogen administration. Paradoxical vasoconstrictor responses to acetylcholine infusion have been demonstrated in the coronary arteries of ovariectomized monkeys fed an atherogenic diet; normal vasodilator responses were restored following either chronic (3 months) (56) or short-term (20 minutes) (60) estrogen administration. Similar restitution of normal coronary vasomotor responses to acetylcholine have been reported in postmenopausal women following short-term administration of ethinyl estradiol (61).

Estrogen also inhibits atherosclerosis by inhibiting the growth and proliferation of VSMCs. VSMC proliferation is an integral part of the atherosclerotic process. Atherosclerosis appears to be initiated by injury to the vessel wall that can be due to a variety of factors, including hyperlipidemia, oxidative stress, hypertension, vessel disruption due to bypass surgery or balloon catheters (62). VSMCs, which normally have a contractile phenotype, change to a secretory phenotype after injury. In the secretory phase, the VSMCs manufacture and secrete extracellular matrix (collagen and elastin), which reduces the effective lumen of the vessel involved. Estrogen-mediated inhibition of atherosclerosis was first demonstrated by Stamler, Pick and Katz in cholesterol-fed chicks over 40 years ago (63). Estrogen can also inhibit the growth of VSMCs in culture (64, 65) and the proliferation of VSMCs in atherosclerotic lesions (66–69).

Balloon injury of the arteries of animals (including rabbit, fowl, swine, and primates) is widely used as an experimental model for the early injury phase of atherosclerosis (70). In this model, inflation of the balloon denudes endothelium and induces a high reproducible intimal migration/proliferation of VSMCs over the entire length of the affected vessel. These studies have provided experimental evidence that estrogen inhibits VSMC proliferation after balloon injury of an artery. Estrogen inhibits neointimal formation (VSMC proliferation and extracellular matrix formation) after balloon injury of the common and external iliac arteries of rabbits (71). Further, our laboratory has shown that myointimal proliferation after balloon injury of the carotid artery is reduced in intact female

Sprague-Dawley rats compared to age matched males and that this sexual dimorphism is dependent on estrogen rather than testosterone (72). This study also showed that physiologic levels of exogenous estrogen can prevent neointimal formation in damaged vessels of gonadectomized rats of both sexes (Figure 2.9). 17β-estradiol inhibited the myointimal response to balloon injury by −60%, an effect comparable to results observed with a variety of other antiproliferative agents in the rat carotid injury model. Using the carotid injury model of Lindner (73), gonadectomy has been shown to enhance, and physiologic levels of 17β-estradiol replacement to suppress, subintimal hyperproliferation in vessels damaged by repetitive passage of angioplasty wires in female mice, thus confirming our observation in the rat (74). In contrast, neither endogenous nor exogenous testosterone at physiologic levels affected neointima formation in the rat carotid injury model (72). We are currently extending these findings by evaluating the effects of progestins, alone and in combination with estrogen, on neointima formation in the rat carotid injury model. Preliminary data suggest that progestins reduce the beneficial effects of 17β-estradiol on neointima formation after balloon injury but have no independent effect on hyperproliferative response to endothelial denudation (75).

The swine model of coronary artery injury by balloon dilation offers advantages over rodent models in that the coronary anatomy, lipid metabolism, vascular cell biology and coagulation profile of the pig are similar to the human (76, 77). Our laboratory is currently examining the effects of exogenous estrogen on neointima formation after balloon injury of swine coronary arteries. Preliminary results indicate that 17β-estradiol administered subcutaneously from sustained release pellets reduces neointima formation in both male and female pigs (78) and that the magnitude of this effect is related to circulating estrogen levels.

In summary, postmenopausal hormone replacement therapy with unopposed estrogen or estrogen plus a progestin appears to afford important protection against the development of atherosclerotic vascular disease via effects on lipids and lipid metabolism, as well as direct effects on the vasculature. These cardiovascular benefits are offset by increased risk of endometrial hyperplasia/carcinoma and of breast cancer, although the magnitude of the breast cancer risk is much debated (79, 80). One solution to this problem may be the development of the selective estrogen receptor modulators (SERMs), a class of compounds with estrogenic effects on vascular tissue and bone and antiestrogenic or neutral effects on breast and uterine tissue (81, 82). The SERMs may protect the vasculature and bone of postmenopausal women without exposing them to excess risk of cancer. Until these compounds become available, postmenopausal estrogen replacement therapy, with or without accompanying progestin, should be considered for all postmenopausal women. In considering whether or not to

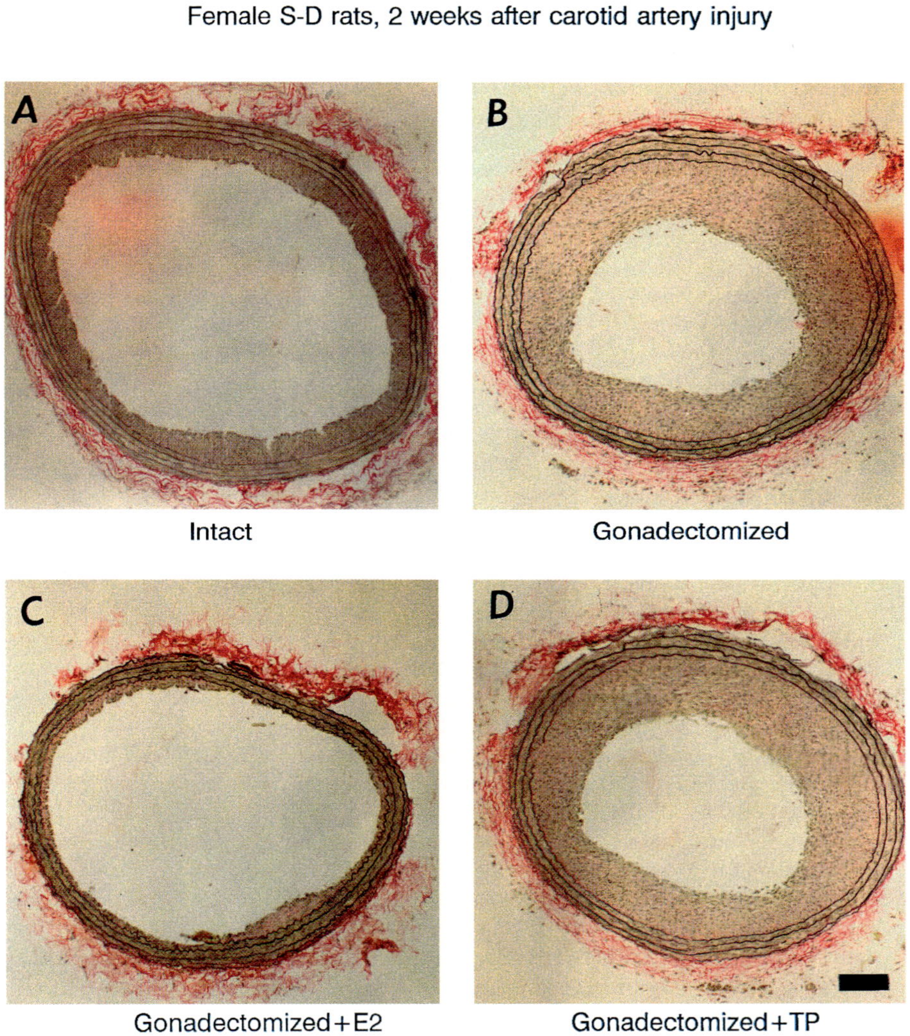

Figure 2.9: Representative light micrographs of right common carotid arteries from female Sprague-Dawley rats 14 days after balloon injury. Balloon-injured right carotid arteries from 1) an intact female rat (A); 2) a gonadectomized female rat (B); 3) a gonadectomized + 17β-estradiol-treated female rat (C) and 4) a gonadectomized + testosterone-treated female rat (D). Magnification × 100, bar = 100 μm. Reproduced from reference 72 with permission.

use postmenopausal hormone replacement therapy, women and their physicians must weigh its beneficial effects on risk of heart disease and osteoporosis against its adverse effects on risk of breast and uterine cancer (40). Because heart disease is so much more common than breast cancer, the impact of post-menopausal hormone replacement therapy on lives saved by decreasing fatal heart attack rates is far greater than on lives lost by increasing breast cancer rates. However, relative risks of cardiovascular disease vs. breast cancer vary greatly among women, so decisions about postmenopausal hormone replacement therapy should be individualized (40).

References

1. Godsland IF, Wynn V, Crook D, Miller NE. Sex, plasma lipoproteins, and atherosclerosis: Prevailing assumptions and outstanding questions. Am Heart J 1987; 114: 1467−1503.
2. Bush TL, Barrett-Connor E. Noncontraceptive estrogen use and cardiovascular disease. Epidemiol Rev 1985; 7: 89−104.
3. 1996 Heart and Stroke Facts Statistics. Dallas: American Heart Association, 1996.
4. Lobo RA. Cardiovascular disease in women: Influence of hormonal replacement therapy. In: Safar M, Stimpel M, Zanchetti A, eds. Hypertension in postmenopausal women. Germany; Springer-Verlag Berlin Heidelberg 1994; 27−44.
5. Knopp RH. The effects of postmenopausal estrogen therapy on the incidence of arteriosclerotic vascular disease. Obstet Gynecol 1988; 72: 23S−30S.
6. Riedel M, Rafflenbeul W, Lichtlen P. Ovarian sex steroids and atherosclerosis. Clin Invest 1993; 71: 406−412.
7. Rich-Edwards JW, Manson JE, Hennekens CH, Buring JE. The primary prevention of coronary heart disease in women. N Engl J Med 1995; 332: 1758−1766.
8. Willett WC, Green A, Stampfer MJ, et al. Relative and absolute excess risks of coronary heart disease among women who smoke cigarettes. N Engl J Med 1987; 317: 1303−1309.
9. Rosenberg L, Palmer JR, Shapiro S. Decline in the risk of myocardial infarction among women who stop smoking. N Engl J Med 1990; 322: 213−217.
10. Burt VL, Whelton P, Roccella EJ, et al. Prevalence of hypertension in the US adult population. Results from the Third National Health and Nutrition Examination Survey. 1988−1991. Hypertension 1995; 25: 305−313.
11. Staessen J, Bulpitt CJ, Fagard K, Lijinen P, Amery A. The influence of menopause on blood pressure. J Human Hypertension 1989; 3: 427−433.
12. Weiss NS. Relationship of menopause to serum cholesterol and arterial pressure: The United States Health Examination Survey of Adults. Am J Epidemiol 1972; 96: 237.
13. Matthews KA, Meilahn E, Kuller LH, Kelsey SF, Caggiula AW, Wing RR. Menopause and risk factors for coronary heart disease. N Engl J Med 1989; 321: 641−646.
14. Hjörtland MC, McNamara PM, Kannel WB. Some atherogenic concomitants of menopause: The Framingham Study. Am J. Epidemiol 1976; 103: 304−311.
15. van Berensteyn EC, van t Hof MA, De Waard H. Contributions of ovarian failure and aging to blood pressure in normotensive perimenopausal women: A mixed longitudinal study. Am J Epidemiol 1989; 129: 947−955.
16. Sempos CT, Cleeman JI, Carroll MD, et al. Prevalence of high blood cholesterol among US adults. An update based on guidelines from the second report of the National Cholesterol Education Program Adult Treatment Panel. JAMA 1993; 269: 3009−3014.
17. Jacobs DR Jr, Meban IL, Bangdiwala SI, Criqui MH, Tyroler HA. High density lipoprotein cholesterol as a predictor of cardiovascular disease mortality in men and women: The follow-up study of the Lipid Research Clinics Prevalence Study. Am J Epidemiol 1990; 131: 32−47.
18. Brunner D, Weisbort J, Meshulam N, et al. Relation of serum total cholesterol and high-density lipoprotein cholesterol percentage to the incidence of definite coronary events: Twenty-year follow-up of the Donolo-Tel Aviv prospective coronary artery disease study. Am J Cardiol 1987; 59: 1271−1276.

19. Oparil S. Cardiovascular risk reduction in women. J Women's Health 1996; 5: 23–32.
20. Gordon DJ, Probstfield JL, Garrison RJ, et al. High-density lipoprotein cholesterol and cardiovascular disease; four prospective American studies. Circulation 1989; 79: 8–15.
21. Crouse JR III. Gender, lipoproteins, diet, and cardiovascular risk: sauce for the goose may not be sauce for the gander. Lancet 1989; 2: 318–320.
22. Barrett-Connor EL, Cohn BA, Wingard DL, Edelstein SL. Why is diabetes mellitus a stronger risk factor for fatal ischemic heart disease in women than in men? The Rancho Bernardo Study. JAMA 1991; 265: 627–631.
23. Manson JE, Colditz GA, Stampfer MJ, et al. A prospective study of maturity-onset diabetes mellitus and risk of coronary heart disease and stroke in women. Arch Intern Med 1991; 151: 1141–1147.
24. Wenger NK. Hypertension and other cardiovascular risk factors in women. Am J Hypertens 1995; 8: 94S–99S.
25. Eaker ED, Castelli WP. Coronary heart disease and its risk factors among women in the Framingham Study. In: Baker ED, Packard B, Wenger NK, Clarkson TB, Tyroler HA, eds. Coronary Heart Disease in Women. Haymarket Doyma Inc, New York, NY, 1987: 122–130.
26. Kleinman JC, Donahue RP, Harris MI, et al. Mortality among diabetics in a national sample. Am J Epidemiol 1988; 128: 389–401.
27. Pan W-H, Cedres LB, Liu K, et al. Relationship of clinical diabetes and asymptomatic hyperglycemia to risk of coronary heart disease mortality in men and women. Am J Epidemiol 1986; 123: 504–516.
28. Walden CE, Knopp RH, Wahl PW, et al. Sex differences in the effect of diabetes mellitus on lipoprotein triglyceride and cholesterol concentrations. N Engl J Med 1984; 311: 953–959.
29. Barrett-Connor E, Witztum JL, Holdbrook M. A community study of high-density lipoproteins in adult non-insulin-dependent diabetics. Am J Epidemiol 1983; 117: 186–192.
30. Evans DJ, Hoffmann RG, Kalkhoff RK, et al. Relationship of androgenic activity to body fat topography, fat cell morphology, and metabolic aberrations in premenopausal women. J Clin Endocrinol Metab 1983; 57: 304–310.
31. Peiris AN, Sothmann MS, Hennes MI, et al. Relative contribution of obesity and body fat distribution to alterations in glucose insulin homeostasis: predictive values of selected indices in premenopausal women. Am J Clin Nutrition 1989; 49: 758–764.
32. Ostlund RE Jr, Staten M, Kohrt WM, Schultz J, Malley M. The ratio of waist-to-hip circumference, plasma insulin level, and glucose intolerance as independent predictors of the HDL_2 cholesterol level in older adults. N Engl J Med 1990; 322: 229–234.
33. Kissebah AH, Evans DJ, Peiris A, Wilson CR. Endocrine characteristics in regional obesities: role of sex steroids. In: Vague J, Bjorntorp P, Guy-Grand B, Rebuffe-Scrive M, Vague P, eds. Metabolic Complications of Human Obesities. Elsevier Science Publishing Co Inc, New York, NY, 1985: 115–131.
34. Poretsky L, Kalin MF. The gonadotropic function of insulin. Endocr Rev 1987; 8: 132–141.
35. Kannel WB, Wolf PA, Castelli WP, D'Agostino RB. Fibrinogen and the risk of cardiovascular disease; the Framingham Study. JAMA 1987; 258: 1183–1186.
36. Nabulsi AA, Folsom AR, White A, et al. Association of hormone-replacement therapy with various cardiovascular risk factors in postmenopausal women. N Engl J Med 1993; 328: 1069–1075.
37. Meillahn EN, Kuller LH, Matthews KA, Kiss JE. Hemostatic factors according to menopausal status and use of hormone replacement therapy. Ann Epidemiol 1992; 2: 445–455.
38. Lerner DJ, Kannell WB. Patterns of coronary heart disease morbidity and mortality in the sexes: a 26-year follow-up of the Framingham population. Am Heart J 1986; 111: 383–390.
39. Colditz GA, Willett WC, Stampfer MJ, Rosner B, Speizer FE, Hennekens CH. Menopause and the risk of coronary heart disease in women. N Engl J Med 1987; 316: 1105–1110.

40. Grady D, Rubin SM, Petitti DB, et al. Hormone therapy to prevent disease and prolong life in postmenopausal women. Ann Intern Med 1992; 117: 1016–1037.
41. Barrett-Connor E. Postmenopausal estrogen and prevention. Ann Intern Med 1191; 115: 455–456.
42. PEPI Trial Writing Group. Effects of estrogen or estrogen/progestin regimens on heart disease risk factors in postmenopausal women. The postmenopausal estrogen/progestin interventions (PEPI) trial. JAMA 1995; 3: 199–208.
43. Schaefer EJ, Foster DM, Zech LA, Lindgren FT, Brewer HB Jr, Levy RI. The effects of estrogen administration on plasma lipoprotein metabolism in premenopausal females. J Clin Endocrinol Metab 1983; 57: 262–267.
44. Kovanen PT, Brown MS, Goldstein JL. Increased binding of low density lipoprotein to liver membranes from rats treated with 17 alpha-ethinyl estradiol. J Biol Chem 1979; 254: 11367–11373.
45. Ma PTS, Yamamoto T, Goldstein JL, Brown MS. Increased mRNA for low density lipoprotein receptor in livers of rabbits treated with 17 alpha ethinyl estradiol. Proc Natl Acad Sci USA 1986; 83: 792–796.
46. Walsh BW, Schiff I, Rosner B, Greenberg L, Ravnikar V, Sacks FM. Effects of postmenopausal estrogen replacement on the concentrations and metabolism of plasma lipoproteins. N Engl J Med 1991; 325: 1196–1204.
47. Pfeffer RI, Kurosaki TT, Charlton SK. Estrogen use and blood pressure in later life. Am J Epidemiol 1979; 110: 469–478.
48. Barrett-Connor E, Wingard DL, Criqui MH. Postmenopausal estrogen use and heart disease risk factors in the 1980s; Rancho Bernardo, Calif. revisited. JAMA 1989; 261: 2095–2100.
49. Deeley RG, Tam SP, Archer TK. The effects of estrogen on apolipoprotein synthesis. Can J Biochem Cell Biol 1985; 63: 882–889.
50. Wagner JD, Clarkson TB, St Clair RW, Schwenke DC, Shively CA, Adams MR. Estrogen and progesterone replacement therapy reduces low density lipoprotein accumulation in the coronary arteries of surgically postmenopausal cynomolgus monkeys. J Clin Invest 1991; 88: 1995–2002.
51. Fischer GM, Bashey RI, Rosenbaum H, Lyttle CR. A possible mechanism in arterial wall for mediation of sex difference in atherosclerosis. Exp Mol Pathol 1985; 43: 288–296.
52. Alexander JJ, Hoenig M, Graham D, Imbembo AL. The effect of estrogen on low-density lipoprotein binding kinetics in aortic endothelial cells. Surgery 1989; 106: 386–391.
53. Rifici VA, Khachandurian AK. The inhibition of low-density lipoprotein oxidation by 17β-estradiol. Metabolism 1992; 41: 1110–1114.
54. Gilligan DM, Quyyumi AA, Cannon RO III. Effects of physiological levels of estrogen on coronary vasomotor function in postmenopausal women. Circulation 1994; 89: 2545–2551.
55. Keaney JF Jr, Shwaery GT, Xu A, Nicolosi RJ, Lascalzo J, Foxall TL, Vita JA. 17β-estradiol preserves endothelial vasodilator function and limits low-density lipoprotein oxidation in hypercholesterolemic swine. Circulation 1994; 89: 2251–2259.
56. Williams JK, Adams MR, Klopfenstein HS. Estrogen modulates responses of atherosclerotic coronary arteries. Circulation 1990; 81: 1680–1687.
57. Harder DR, Coulson PB. Estrogen receptors and effects of estrogen on membrane electrical properties of coronary vascular smooth muscle. J Cell Physiol 1979; 100: 375–382.
58. Chang WC, Nakao J, Orimo H, Murota SI. Stimulation of prostaglandin cyclooxygenase and prostacyclinsynthetase activities by estradiol in rat aortic smooth muscle cells. Biochim Biophys Acta 1980; 620: 472–482.
59. Palmer RMJ, Ferrige AG, Moncada S. Nitric oxide release accounts for the biological activity of endothelium-derived relaxing factor. Nature 1987; 327: 524–526.
60. Williams JK, Adams MR, Herrington DM, Clarkson TB. Short-term administration of estrogen and vascular responses of atherosclerotic coronary arteries. J Am Coll Cardiol 1992; 20: 452–457.

61. Reis SE, Gloth ST, Blumenthal RS, Resar JR, Zacur HA, Gerstenblith G, Brinker JA. Ethinyl estradiol acutely attenuates abnormal coronary vasomotor responses to acetylcholine in postmenopausal women. Circulation 1994; 89: 52–60.
62. Ross R. The pathogenesis of atherosclerosis: a perspective for the 1990s. (Review) Nature 1993; 362: 801–809.
63. Stamler J, Pick R, Katz LN. Prevention of coronary atherosclerosis by estrogen-androgen administration in the cholesterol-fed chick. Circ Res 1953; 1: 94–98.
64. Vargas R, Wroblewska B, Rego A, Hatch J, Ramwell PW. Oestradiol inhibits smooth muscle cell proliferation of pig coronary artery. Br J Pharmacol 1993; 109: 612–617.
65. Fischer-Dzoga K, Wissler RW, Vesselinovitch D. The effect of estradiol on the proliferation of rabbit aortic medial tissue culture cells induced by hyperlipemic serum. Exper Mol Pathol 1983; 39: 355–363.
66. Moskowitz MS, Moskiwitz AA, Bradford WL, Wissler RW. Changes in serum lipids and coronary arteries of the rat in response to estrogens. Arch Pathol 1956; 61: 245–263.
67. Constantinides P, Gutmann-Auersperg N, Hospes D, Williams K. Estradiol and prednisone in rabbit atherosclerosis. Arch Pathol 1962; 73: 277–280.
68. Rhee CY, Spaet TH, Temerman MB, Lajam F, Shiang HH. Estrogen suppression of surgically induced vascular intimal hyperplasia in rabbits. J Lab Clin Med 1977; 90: 77–84.
69. Foegh ML, Khirabadi BS, Nakanishi T, Vargas R, Ramwell PW. Estradiol protects against experimental cardiac transplant atherosclerosis. Transplant 1987; 19: 90–95.
70. Muller DWM, Ellis SG, Topol EJ. Experimental models of coronary artery restenosis. J Am Coll Cardiol 1992; 19: 418–432.
71. Foegh M. Asotra S, Howell M, Ramwell P. Estradiol inhibition of arterial neointimal hyperplasia after balloon injury. J Vasc Surg 1994; 19: 722–726.
72. Chen SJ, Li H, Durand J, Oparil S. Chen YF. Estrogen reduces myointimal proliferation after balloon injury of rat carotid artery. Circulation 1996; 93: 577–584.
73. Lindner V, Fingerle J, Reidy MA. Mouse model of arterial injury. Circ Res 1993; 73: 792–796.
74. Sullivan TR Jr, Karas RH, Aronovitz M, Faller GT, Ziar JP, Smith JJ, O'Donnell TF, Mendelsohn ME. Estrogen inhibits the response-to-injury in a mouse carotid artery model. J Clin Invest 1995; 96: 2482–2488.
75. Levine RL, Chen SJ, Durand J, Chen YF, Oparil S. 17β-estradiol but not medroxyprogesterone inhibits neointima formation after balloon injury of rat carotid arteries. J Invest Med 1996; 44: 26A.
76. Schwartz RS, Murphy JG, Edwards WD, Camrud AR, Viestra RE, Holmes DR. Restenosis after balloon angioplasty. A practical proliferative model porcine coronary arteries. Circulation 1990; 82: 2190–2200.
77. Steele PM, Chesebro JH, Stanson A, Holmes DR Jr, Dewanjee MK, Badimon L, Fuster V. Balloon angioplasty. Natural history of the pathophysiological response to injury in a pig model. Circ Res 1985; 57: 105–112.
78. Levine RL, Anderson PG, Lyle K, Yadav SS, Oparil S, Roubin GS. 17-β estradiol inhibits restenosis after coronary angioplasty in pigs. J Invest Med 1996; 44: 26A.
79. Colditz GA, Hankinson SE, Hunter DJ, et al. The use of estrogens and progestins and the risk of breast cancer in postmenopausal women. N Engl J Med 1995; 332: 1589–1593.
80. Stanford JL, Colditz GA. Controversies in science; Hormone replacement therapy. The benefits of hormone replacement therapy outweigh the breast-cancer risks for some women – The benefits of hormone replacement therapy do not outweigh the increased risk of breast cancer. J NIH Research 1996; 8: 40–41.
81. Kauffman RF, Bryant HU. Selective estrogen receptor modulators. Drug News and Perspectives. 1995; 8: 531–539.
82. Black LJ, Sato M, Rowley ER, et al. Raloxifene (LY139481) prevents bone loss and reduces serum cholesterol without causing uterine hypertrophy in ovariectomized rats. J Clin Invest 1194; 93: 63–69.

3 The epidemiology of menopause and associated cardiovascular disease

Jan A. Staessen, Leszek Bieniaszewski, Ivo Brosens, Robert Fagard

Introduction

The climacteric is a normal aging phenomenon in women and consists of the gradual transition from the reproductive to the non-reproductive phase of life. The menopause is usually defined as the cessation of menstruation or as the last menstrual period and marks the end of ovulation. Ovarian failure following the menopause is characterized by estrogen deficiency. Estrogens may exert a protective effect on the cardiovascular system, for instance by increasing the ratio of high density (HDL) to low density lipoproteins (HDL) in plasma or by inhibiting arterial vasomotion and thrombosis.

This short article reviews the epidemiology of menopause and its alleged association with cardiovascular disease, in particular hypertension and coronary heart disease. A detailed account of the reviewed studies, including a full reference list, has been published elsewhere (1).

Menopause

There is striking concordance in the literature that in Western industrialized societies the median age at the menopause is currently around 50 years. In non-caucasian women, however, the menopause seems to occur earlier. American and South African black women have an earlier menopause than their white counterparts. Moreover, malnutrition and low body weight are associated with a precocious menopause.

The most important factor determining a woman's age at the menopause is the number of ovarian follicles. Human primordial germ cells separate from the somatic cells at an early stage of embryogenesis. Some 1000 to 2000 migrate to the gonadal ridge, where they rapidly multiply up to 5 to 7 million follicles around the fifth month of intra-uterine life. Thereafter, multiplication ceases and the primordial follicles commence to dissolve, so that at birth both fetal ovaries combined contain no more than about 2 million follicles. This number continues to fall after birth. Fewer than 0.02% of the follicles present at birth are ovulated during the reproductive phase of life, while the remainder degenerates. In the immediate premenopausal period, the rate of loss of primordial follicles accelerates, and menopause intervenes when the number of follicles has fallen below a critical number.

Nulliparous women tend to have an earlier menopause, while increased parity, particularly in higher social classes, is associated with a later menopause. Mothers of twins enter the menopause about 1 year earlier than women who have only had singleton infants. Women whose last pregnancy occurred before the age of 28 probably have an earlier menopause than those with their last pregnancy at a later age. Women who smoke enter the menopause up to 2 years earlier than those who do not. The effects of smoking on menopausal age seem to be dose-related and may be mediated in part via a lowered estrogen production and/or via toxic substances in the tobacco smoke, which may contribute to the premature destruction of the primordial oocytes.

By the year 2025, 23% of the population will be aged 60 or over. As a result of the increasing life expectancy in the first and second worlds, many women will be postmenopausal for over one-third of their lives. Already now, approximately 95% of all women living in industrialized countries experience menopause during their life-time. These numbers help to explain why over the past decades menopause has grown from a subject that was peripheral to medical interest into one which takes a central place in clinical practice.

Hypertension

Systolic pressure increases with age at least until the eighth decade of life, whereas diastolic pressure rises only until 50 years of age. Following middle-age, both systolic and diastolic blood pressure become higher in women than in men, whereas the reverse is true in the first half of life. This observation suggests that ovarian failure and the ensuing estrogen deficiency may influence the age-related increase in blood pressure in women. However, the blood pressure changes associated with menopause are difficult to evaluate, because menopause coincides with aging, and because both menopause and blood pressure are influenced by common factors, such as body mass index, socio-economic class and smoking.

Taylor et al. (2) were among the first to contrast the prevalence of hypertension in menopausal women and office workers. They found that hypertension was no more prevalent among a group of 179 castrated women and 21 women with natural menopause than in the control subjects and that "vasomotor instability," as exhibited by hot flushes, perspiration and tachycardia, was not necessarily associated with hypertension. The conclusion from this pioneering study (2) was that the relationship between hypertension and menopause was incidental and that the loss of ovarian secretion was neither a primary nor a contributory cause of arterial hypertension.

In Belgium, the association between menopause and systolic and diastolic blood pressure was explored in a random sample of 278 pre- and 184 postmenopausal women, who were from 35 to 59 years old (3). All women were participants in a cross-sectional population survey with a sample size of 3950 eligible persons, of whom 67% took part. All women were characterized by the average of 10 blood pressure readings, i. e. 5 consecutive readings in the sitting position obtained at each of 2 separate home visits. The postmenopausal women had higher systolic (132 vs. 121 mmHg), diastolic (81 vs. 75 mmHg) and pulse (51 vs. 46 mmHg) pressures than the premenopausal subjects (Figure 3.1). Hypertension was more frequently observed following menopause (40 vs 10%; $p < 0.001$). After stratification by age and body mass index, the odds of having hypertension in premenopausal as compared with postmenopausal women were 2.2 (95% confidence interval [CI]: 1.1 to 4.4; $p = 0.03$). After adjustment of blood pressure for significant covariates, such as body mass index, pulse rate and the intake of estrogens and/or progestogens, the slope of systolic pressure

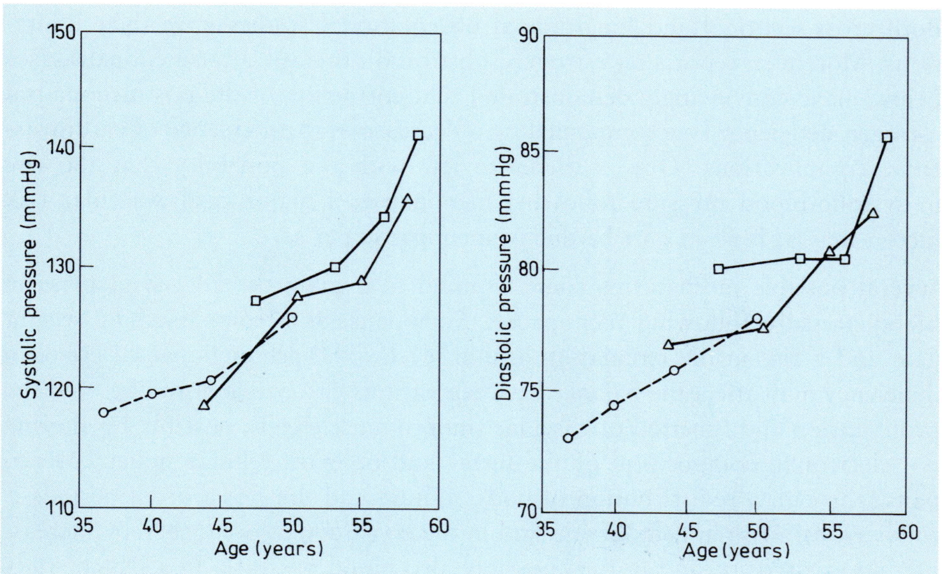

Figure 3.1: Systolic (left panel) and diastolic (right panel) blood pressures in fourths of the age distribution in premenopausal women (○, n = 278), and in women with natural (□, n = 120) and surgical (△, n = 64) menopause. From Staessen et al. (3); with permission.

on age was 0.5 mmHg per year steeper in the post- than in the premenopausal women. The relation of diastolic pressure with age had the same slope among pre- and postmenopausal subjects, but in postmenopausal women the regression line was shifted upward by 2.3 mmHg ($p = 0.03$).

Several other cross-sectional and longitudinal studies have addressed the alleged association between hypertension and menopause (Table 3.1). On balance, the longitudinal surveys suggest that menopause per se is not associated with an increase in blood pressure and a greater incidence of hypertension. The results from the cross-sectional studies are more equivocal, as some surveys have found a positive association and other studies no relation. Although longitudinal studies are often considered to be superior to cross-sectional surveys, both are open to confounding. Cross-sectional designs may preclude the accurate assessment of changes over time, which are due to differences in growth or development across generations (cohort differences). Longitudinal surveys, on the other hand, are easily confounded by effects related to the time of measurement. Changes in the environmental conditions inevitably occur over a given period of follow-up, and may lead to an over- or under-estimation of the true intra-individual changes and relationships over time. In particular, clinical, biochemical and technical measurements may be unduely influenced by the unavoidable renewal of chemicals, standards, and instrumentation, or changes in the team of observers.

Both cross-sectional and longitudinal observational studies have their limitations. Moreover, reports on estrogen substitution therapy after menopause (see below) have convincingly demonstrated that correction of the postmenopausal estrogen deficiency is accompanied by a decrease in the incidence of cardiovascular complications. One is therefore left with the possibilty that the rise in systolic blood pressure following menopause, a major cardiovascular risk factor, may at least in part be due to menopause per se.

Several possible mechanisms come to mind to explain the alleged increase in blood pressure following menopause. Menopause is accompanied by weight gain and a rise in the circulating insulin levels. The postmenopausal estrogen deficiency may affect the balance between various vasoactive hormones and the proliferation and function of vascular smooth muscle cells, possibly by altering the electrolyte composition of the intra- and/or extra-cellular milieu. Menopause through a redistribution of body sodium and the cessation of periods is followed by a rise in hemoglobin and in the erythrocyte count, thereby increasing blood viscosity, and in turn possibly also blood pressure. In a Dutch study (4) menopause has also been found to be associated with calcification of the abdominal aorta. After adjustment for age and other cardiovascular risk indicators, women with natural menopause had a 3.4 times greater risk of having

Table 3.1: The association between menopause and blood pressure in various studies.

Study[a]	Type of menopause[b]	Adjustments[c]	ΔSBP#	ΔDBP#	HT#
Longitudinal studies					
Hjortland et al., 1976	N (480) vs. P (3,117)	MT, A	−0.8[d]	−0.2[d]	
	H (77) vs. P (3,117)	MT, A	−0.3[d]	+1.4[d]	
	C (137) vs. P (3,117)	MT, A	−0.1[d]	−0.6[d]	
Lindquist, 1982	N (343) vs. P (324)	A	−1.1[d]	−1.0[d]	
	N (343) vs. P (304)	A	+0.1[d]	+0.9[d]	
van Berensteyn et al., 1989	N (168)	A	−1.3[e]	−0.6[e]	
van Berensteyn et al., 1992	N (37)	BMI, IA, IBP, IBMI	−0.7[e]	−0.1[e]	
	N (139)	BMI, IA, IBP, IBMI	−0.7[e]	−0.2[e]	
	N (63)	BMI, IA, IBP, IBMI	+1.1[e]	−0.3[e]	
Cross-sectional studies					
Weiss, 1972	N (297, S (172), P (428)	A	+4.7[d]	+2.7[d]	
Lindquist and Bengtsson, 1980	N (162) vs. P (164), 50 years old	A	−5.0[d]	0[d]	
	N (681) vs. P (728), other ages		−5.4[d]	−1.1[d]	
Eferakeya and Imasuen, 1986	N (287) vs. P (252)	A, SEC	+16.1[d]	+15.7[d]	
Staessen et al., 1989	N & S (120 & 64) vs. P (278)	A, AHT, BMI, EP, PR	+0.5[f]	+2.5[d]	+30 (>140/>90)[d]
Wu et al., 1990	N (176) vs. P (422)	A	+2.9[d]	−0.1[d]	+8 (>140/>90)[d]
Other designs					
Taylor et al., 1947	N & C (21 & 179) vs. OW (2,860)				−1 (>149/>94)[d]

[a] Studies are identified by the first author, year of publication; full identification of all studies is available in reference 1.

[b] Groups considered in the analysis: C = castrated women (bilateral oophorectomy); H = women who underwent hysterectomy not combined with bilateral oophorectomy; N = women with natural menopause; OW = office workers; P = premenopausal (control) subjects; S = women who underwent surgical menopause. In parentheses: number of patients.

[c] A = age; AHT = antihypertensive treatment; BMI = body mass index; EP = intake of estrogens and/or progestogens; IA = initial age; IBP = initial blood pressure; IBMI = initial body mass index; MT = measurement technique; PR = pulse rate; SEC = socio-economic class.

[d] ΔSBP, ΔDBP = change in systolic, diastolic pressure (mmHg) taken directly from the publications or calculated according to the published results with weighting by number, if the published articles included more than 1 group; HT = difference in the prevalence of hypertension (%) as defined by the systolic/diastolic blood pressure criteria (mmHg) given between parentheses.

[e] ΔSBP, ΔDBP = age-related changes in systolic, diastolic pressure (mmHg/year) in various groups of menopausal women.

[f] ΔSBP, ΔDBP = difference in the slope of systolic pressure on age associated with menopause.

atherosclerosis of the abdominal aorta than premenopausal subjects (CI: 1.2 to 9.7; $p < 0.05$), and women with surgical menopause a 5.5 greater risk (CI: 1.9 to 15.8; $p < 0.005$). Stiffening of the large arteries after menopause may explain why, as observed in the Belgian survey (3), the slope of systolic pressure on age steepened and the pulse pressure widened in the postmenopausal subjects.

Other cardiovascular diseases

In premenopausal women, the prevalence and incidence of cardiovascular diseases is lower than in middle-aged men. The cardiovascular risk of women rises after the age of 50, although even in postmenopausal women, the incidence of fatal and non-fatal cardiovascular complications combined still remains nearly 45% lower than in age-matched male subjects. Nevertheless, in absolute numbers, more women than men die from cardiovascular illnesses at an older age, because the aged female population at risk is substantially larger than the male.

The relationship between menopause and cardiovascular disease, in particular ischemic heart disease, has been examined in several studies, most of which (5–7), but not all (8), found that the age-adjusted rates rose after menopause (for additional studies, see reference 1). The Nurses' Health Study (9) included 121,700 American women from 30 to 55 years old, who were followed from 1976 to 1982. In this prospective cohort study (9), the relationship between menopause and the risk of coronary heart disease was studied. Information on menopausal status, the type of menopause, and other risk factors was first collected in 1976 and updated every 2 years by mailing questionnaires. Through 1982, the follow-up rate was 98% for mortality and 95% for non-fatal events. After adjustment for age and cigarette smoking, women who had undergone a natural menopause and who had never taken estrogen replacement therapy, had no appreciable increase in the risk of coronary heart disease, as compared with premenopausal women (adjusted rate ratio: 1.2; CI: 0.8 to 1.8). Again compared with premenopausal women, the occurrence of a natural menopause together with the use of estrogens did not affect the coronary risk (rate ratio: 0.8; CI: 0.4 to 1.3). By contrast, women who had undergone bilateral oophorectomy and who had never taken estrogens after menopause had an increased risk (rate ratio: 2.2; CI: 1.2 to 4.2). However, the use of estrogens in the postmenopausal period appeared to eliminate this augmented risk as compared with the premenopausal subjects (rate ratio: 0.9; CI: 0.6 to 1.6). This large cohort study (9) therefore suggested that, by contrast to natural menopause, bilateral oophorectomy raised the risk of coronary heart disease, but that this increased risk could be reversed by estrogen replacement therapy. On the other hand, the findings of the Nurses' Health Study were gathered in a highly educated and health conscious professional group and should therefore not necessarily be applicable to the population at large.

Several lines of evidence suggest that, in addition to the aging process, menopause may be involved in explaining the higher cardiovascular morbidity and mortality in post- compared with premenopausal subjects. Estrogens directly influence several cardiovascular risk factors, such as body mass index and blood viscosity, but the greatest weight is usually attached to the changes in the serum lipid and lipoprotein concentrations (10, 11). In general, estrogens raise the serum level of HDL cholesterol, especially the HDL_2 subfraction, and lower the serum concentration of LDL cholesterol. Usually, estrogens also produce a slight decrease in serum total cholesterol. These are the theoretically desirable changes cited most frequently to support the epidemiological findings pertaining to estrogen deficiency and cardiovascular disease. Oral estrogens also elevate serum triglyceride concentrations, but this is not considered to be an important adverse effect (11).

Retrospective evidence from case-control and other studies of postmenopausal women treated with estrogens, mostly unopposed conjugated equine estrogens, in general support, or at least do not contradict, the concept of a cardioprotective effect of estrogen (Table 3.2). In many of the case-control studies relatively few women treated with estrogens were included (16% on average) and the duration of treatment was short (15 months). These factors probably explain why the benefit of estrogen replacement therapy was significant in only one (12) of the case-control studies. By contrast, most of the prospective, but non-randomized, cohort studies of estrogen therapy in postmenopausal women indicate a clear benefit in terms of coronary artery disease and show a lower mortality from coronary and cardiovascular complications (Table 3.2).

Conclusions

Menopause, i. e. the end of menstruation, constitutes an important physiological and psychological change in a women's life time and usually takes place around 50 years of age. Systematic interest in the menopause by physicians arose in the middle of the last century, at a time when the interest in the care of "the diseases of women" grew exponentially. However, it was not until the last decades of the 20th century that the postmenopausal years became generally recognized as a phase of the female life cycle, which in some of its aspects may benefit from medical intervention.

Despite these new insights, it remains extremely difficult to disentangle the effects of aging and menopause per se on the cardiovascular system, on the recognized cardiovascular risk indicators, and on the prevalence and incidence

Table 3.2: The association between hormone replacement therapy and ischemic heart disease.

Study[a]	Cases[b]	Relative risk[c]
Case-control studies		
Adam et al., 1981	76 (151)	E: 0.7
Bain et al., 1981	123 (2,460)	C: 0.7, E: 0.9
Jick et al., 1978	17 (34)	C: 7.5
Pfeffer et al., 1978	196 (520)	C: 0.8, E: 0.9
Szklo et al., 1984	39 (45)	E: 0.6
Rosenberg et al., 1976	366 (6,830)	C: 1.0
Rosenberg et al., 1980	447 (1,832)	C: 1.3, F: 1.2
Ross et al., 1981	133 (266)	vs. living controls – E: 0.4 <> vs. death controls – E: 0.6
Thompson et al., 1989	603 (1,206)	E: 1.4[d]
Cohort studies		
Bush et al., 1987	50 (2,270)	fatal CHD – C: 0.4
Burch et al., 1974	9 (737)	fatal CHD – C: 0.4
Criqui et al., 1988	87 (1,868)	fatal CHD – 0.8
Hammond et al., 1979	58 (610)	CHD – C: 0.3
Henderson et al., 1991	149 (8,841)	fatal MI – C: 0.6 <> fatal CHD – C: 0.8
Hunt et al., 1987	20 (4,544)	fatal CHD – C: 0.5
Petitti et al., 1979	26 (16,759)	MI – C: 1.2
Petitti et al., 1986	37 (16,638)	fatal CVD – E: 0.5
Stampfer et al., 1985	90 (32,317)	fatal and non-fatal CHD – C: 0.3, E: 0.5
Stampfer et al., 1991	205 (48,470)	CHD – C: 0.6, F: 0.8 <> fatal CVD – C: 0.6, F: 0.8
Wilson et al., 1985	48 (1,234)	CHD – C: 1.9 <> fatal CVD – C: 1.9

[a] Studies are identified by the first author and year of publication; full identification of all studies is available in reference 1.

[b] Number of cases. The number of controls or the total number subjects enrolled in the cohort studies is presented between parentheses.

[c] The risk of ischemic heart disease among women who received estrogen replacement therapy vs. women who did not; C = risk ratio for users vs. non-users or never users; E = risk ratio for ever users vs. never users; F = risk ratio for former users vs. never users.
Abbreviations: CHD = coronary heart disease; CVD = cardiovascular disease; MI = myocardial infarction.

[d] Strokes (n = 244) and myocardial infarctions (n = 359) were combined.

of cardiovascular illnesses, such as hypertension and coronary heart disease. For instance, epidemiological observations on their own could not establish with certainty that menopause is independently associated with a raised cardiovascular risk. This became only unambiguously clear after the cohort studies (Table 3.2) had overwhelmingly demonstrated that estrogen replacement therapy is accompanied by a decrease in overall mortality, which is principally mediated through a beneficial effect on the incidence and fatality rate of coronary heart disease. The protective effect of exogenous estrogens in postmenopausal women strongly suggests that ovarian failure, in its own right, must constitute a cardiovascular risk factor. Estrogen deficiency may principally, albeit not exclusively, operate trough its influence on the lipid metabolism.

The influence of menopause per se on blood pressure, another major cardiovascular risk factor in older persons, remains uncertain. The cohort studies do not support a direct influence of menopause on the incidence of hypertension and the evidence from the cross-sectional studies is equivocal. Nevertheless, there is some suggestion that estrogen replacement treatment may reduce the incidence of stroke (13). One may therefore envisage the possibility that observational studies with more bias free methods to measure the blood pressure than conventional sphygmomanometry, such as ambulatory monitoring, as well as further studies with estrogen replacement therapy, will tilt the allegedly positive association between menopause and blood pressure elevation above the horizon of epidemiological visibility.

Acknowledgements

Epidemiological research relevant to this review article has been supported by the International Lead Zinc Research Organization (Research Triangle Park, North Carolina, USA), the Province of Limburg (Hasselt, Belgium), the municipalities Hechtel-Eksel and Lommel (Belgium), the National Fund for Medical Research, the Incentive Program *'Health Hazards'* (Science Policy Office, Prime Minister's Services), the Ministry of the Flemish Community (Department of Labor and Social Affairs), Astra Pharmaceuticals Inc, Bristol-Meyers-Squibb Inc. (all in Brussels, Belgium) and Schwarz Pharma AG (Monheim, Germany).

References

1. Staessen JA, Bieniaszewski L, Brosens I, Fagard R. The epidemiology of menopause and its association with cardiovascular disease. in Messerli F (ed): Hypertension and Other Cardiovascular Risk Factors After the Menopause. New York, Marcel Dekker Inc. 1995; pp 43–78.
2. Taylor RD, Corcoron AC, Page IH. Menopausal hypertension: a critical study. Am J Med Sci 1947; 213: 475–476.
3. Staessen J, Bulpitt CJ, Fagard R, Lijnen P, Amery A. The influence of menopause on blood pressure. J Hum Hypertens 1989; 3: 427–433.
4. Witteman JCM, Grobbee DE, Kok FJ, Hofman A, Valkenburg HA. Increased risk of atherosclerosis in women after the menopause. Brit Med J 1989; 298: 642–644.
5. Johansson S, Vedin A, Wilhelmsson C. Myocardial infarction in women. Epidemiol Rev 1983; 5: 67–95.
6. Gordon T, Kannel WB, Hjortland MC, McNamara PM. Menopause and coronary heart disease: the Framingham Study. Ann Intern Med 1978; 89: 157–161.
7. Rosenberg L, Hennekens CH, Rosner B, Belanger C, Rothman KJ, Speizer FE. Early menopause and the risk of myocardial infarction. Am J Obstet Gynecol 1981; 139: 47–51.
8. Wilhelmsen L, Bengtsson C, Elmfeldt D, Vedin A, Wilhelmsson C, Tibblin G, Lindqvist O, Wedel H. Multiple risk prediction of myocardial infarction in women as compared with men. Brit Heart J 1977; 39: 1179–1185.

9. Colditz GA, Willett WC, Stampfer MJ, Rosner B, Speizer FE, Hennekens CH. Menopause and the risk of coronary heart disease in women. N Engl J Med 1987; 316: 1105–1110.
10. Lobo RA. Clinical review 27 : effects of hormonal replacement on lipids and lipoproteins in postmenopausal women. J Clin Endocrinol Metab 1991; 73: 925–930.
11. Walsh BW, Schiff I, Rosner B, Greenberg L, Ravnikar V, Sacks FM. Effects of postmenopausal estrogen replacement on the concentrations and metabolism of plasma lipoproteins. N Engl J Med 1991; 325: 1196–1204.
12. Ross RK, Paganini-Hill A, Mack TM, Arthur M, Henderson BE. Menopausal estrogen therapy and protection from death from ischaemic heart disease. Lancet 1981; i: 858–860.
13. Hammond CB, Jelovsek FR, Lee KL, Creasman WT, Parker RT. Effects of long-term estrogen replacement therapy. I. Metabolic effects. Am J Obstet Gynecol 1979; 133: 525–536.

4 Hormone replacement therapy in postmenopausal women: who, why and how long to treat?

John C. Stevenson

Hormone replacement therapy (HRT) consists of oestrogens given as naturally occurring steroids to postmenopausal women in a dose which corrects their oestrogen deficiency and restores levels to those seen in the lower end of the normal premenopausal range. A second steroid, a progestogen, is also included in HRT regimens when appropriate.

Oestrogens

The oestrogens commonly used are oestradiol-17β, oestrone sulphate and conjugated equine oestrogens. The more potent synthetic oestrogens, such as ethinyloestradiol, are not used in modern HRT. Oestrogens will abolish most symptoms which are due to oestrogen deficiency. Side-effects of oestrogens include breast swelling and tenderness, nausea and fluid retention. These side-effects are transient and usually resolve spontaneously after about three months of therapy. They are more common in older women who have been oestrogen deficient for some considerable time, in excess of five years. Such side-effects can be minimized or even prevented by starting older women on low doses of oestrogens and increasing the dose slowly after a few weeks until the desired dose is reached.

Progestogens

If the postmenopausal woman still has an intact uterus, then oestrogen will also stimulate growth of the uterine endometrium. This can lead to erratic bleeding and eventually to endometrial hyperplasia and neoplasia. To circumvent this unwanted effect, a progestogen is given usually in a cyclical fashion. Provided that an adequate dose of progestogen is given for a sufficient time, at least 12 days per month, bleeding is regularised and the increased risk of endometrial carcinoma development seen with oestrogen alone is abolished (1).

Various different progestogen preparations may be used, but these can be broadly divided into 19 nor-testosterone derivatives, such as norgestrel, which have androgenic properties and C-21 steroids, such as dydrogesterone, which are less androgenic. Side-effects from progestogens are much more common than from oestrogens and include breast discomfort, low abdominal pain and bloating, low backache, depression and irritability, and premenstrual-like symptoms. Such side-effects may be abolished by changing the progestogen type, and it is sometimes necessary to try a number of different products before a suitable one is found.

The main drawback to HRT with cyclical progestogen administration is that approximately 90% of women will experience a regular withdrawal bleed around the end of the progestogen course. It should of course be remembered that a withdrawal bleed is not essential for endometrial protection. The bleed is quite predictable once a woman is established on HRT and may diminish with long-term use until it represents only a little spotting. However, bleeding limits the acceptability of HRT in some women, particularly the elderly. Attempts have therefore been made to reduce or even eliminate the bleeding. One approach has been to reduce the frequency of bleeding by giving the progestogen every third month rather than monthly. However, the long-term safety of this approach is not established and there have been concerns that it may not adequately protect the endometrium (2). Another approach is to give the progestogen continuously with the oestrogen, thereby suppressing any endometrial growth and inducing amenorrhoea (3). Such continuous combined HRT seems to be very effective for the skeleton, particularly in elderly women (4), but there are some concerns about the metabolic effects of these treatments which may be less beneficial than with cyclical HRT (5, 6). Thus the overall effect on cardiovascular protection from continuous combined HRT needs to be clarified. Some spotting or bleeding is not uncommon when continuous combined HRT is first initiated but this usually disappears within the first 3 to 6 months. About 25–40% of women fail to achieve amenorrhea, and the treatment should probably be abandoned if bleeding still occurs after six months. An alternative to continuous combined HRT is tibolone, a molecule with oestrogenic, progestogenic and androgenic properties which also does not usually cause bleeding in women who are clearly established as being postmenopausal. Tibolone is also effective in relieving menopause symptoms and preventing postmenopausal bone loss (7), but again it has certain metabolic effects which are potentially undesirable (8).

Routes of administration

Oestrogens have traditionally been given orally, but there is a disadvantage to this route of administration. Following absorption through the stomach and intestine, high levels of steroid are reached in the portal vein giving a bolus effect to the liver – the hepatic first-pass effect. This can result in some potentially unwanted effects of increased hepatic protein (9) and enzyme production, particularly in terms of coagulation factors. Oral oestrogen administration also leads to conversion of oestradiol to oestrone in the gut wall, which leads to an unphysiological oestradiol/oestrone ratio in the circulation. To circumvent these problems, various non-oral routes of administration have been attempted. Oestradiol can be given buccally or sublingually, through the skin as a gel or in a transdermal patch, through the vagina as a cream, tablet or ring, or implanted in the subcutaneous fat as a slow-release pellet. These routes of administration result in a more physiological oestradiol/oestrone ratio. Furthermore, some women regard the use of patches or gels as being a more natural way of taking hormones since they are closer to mimicking normal ovarian function. The advantage of the patches, particularly the matrix patches in which the oestradiol is actually in the plastic matrix, is that they are easy to apply, give fairly constant oestradiol delivery, and need to be changed only once or twice a week depending on the product. The advantage of implants is that they need to be inserted infrequently as they last for six months or more; their drawback is that they cannot be easily removed, and they may lead to a build-up of oestradiol in the blood if they are given too frequently.

Of the progestogens, to date only norethisterone acetate can be administered through a transdermal patch effectively. It has also been incorporated into vaginal rings experimentally. Norgestrel can be given in an intra-uterine device which protects the endometrium without the necessity of systemic absorption of the steroid. Natural progesterone can be given orally and as either pessaries or suppositories. Whilst progesterone may have some metabolic advantages over certain progestogens, side-effects, particularly drowsiness, limit its acceptance.

Indications for HRT

There are currently 3 main indications for giving HRT. These are firstly to relieve symptoms due to oestrogen deficiency, secondly to prevent or treat postmenopausal osteoporosis, and thirdly to prevent or treat coronary heart disease (CHD) in women with established risk.

Oestrogen-deficiency symptoms

The classical menopausal symptoms due to oestrogen deficiency are vasomotor symptoms, particularly hot flushes and night sweats. Some women may also experience migraines with the onset of the menopause, particularly those who suffered from migraine around the time of menstruation premenopausally (menstrual migraine). These symptoms rapidly respond to HRT, with relief occurring sometimes within days of the onset of treatment. Psychological symptoms are also associated with the menopause. Mood swings and irritability are typical, but depression and anxiety may also be related to hormone deficiency. Many patients complain of difficulty with memory and concentration, loss of self confidence, and some experience panic attacks. Whilst symptoms such as these can arise from other causes, it is always worth a symptomatic trial of treatment with HRT in women of appropriate age. A complete lack of effect of HRT given in suitable dosage by 6 months suggests that the symptoms are unconnected with oestrogen deficiency. Genito-urinary tract symptoms arise due to atrophy following the loss of oestrogen at the menopause. Urinary symptoms such as frequency, nocturia, dysuria, urgency and urge incontinence are commonly related to oestrogen deficiency and may respond to oestrogen replacement (10). Vaginal dryness due to atrophic vaginitis will also respond, and topically applied oestrogen may be used for this.

There are many other symptoms arising around the menopause which may occasionally be influenced by HRT even though there is no definitive clinical proof of efficacy. Arthralgia, particularly of small joints may anecdotally respond, and there is some suggestion that HRT may sometimes benefit rheumatoid arthritis. Angina in early postmenopausal women is particularly worthy of mention.

Syndrome X, a condition characterized by angina, positive ECG exercise test or stress thallium scan but no visible abnormality on coronary angiography, is more common in women than in men and frequently arises around the time of menopause. This has suggested that it might in part be hormone-linked. We have found that about 50% of postmenopausal women with syndrome X will actually respond to HRT in terms of ECG exercise test improvement (11).

Symptomatic treatment guidelines

Treatment for any menopause symptoms needs to be given for as long as the symptoms require relief. In the case of symptoms such as hot flushes, 6–12 months may be sufficient since they can be self-limiting. HRT can be withdrawn slowly to see whether or not the symptoms recur. If they do, then a further period of treatment, perhaps for another twelve months, can be undertaken. Other symptoms, such as genitourinary symptoms or angina, may require long-term treatment. The dosage of oestrogen should be titrated according to the clinical response.

Osteoporosis

Osteoporosis is a condition characterized by reduced bone density and loss of skeletal microstructure which results in an increased risk of fragility fractures. The condition is much more common in women than in men due to the effects of the menopause on the skeleton. The eventual development of osteoporosis depends largely on two factors, namely peak bone density and subsequent bone loss. Peak bone density is attained soon after the end of linear skeletal growth, and is largely genetically determined. It is thus not readily amenable to manipulation. Subsequent bone loss in women occurs in relation to loss of ovarian function at the menopause (12). There is a period of fairly rapid bone loss which lasts for 5 to 10 years following the menopause. Thereafter the rate of loss slows but still continues into old age. This loss is predominantly due to increased bone remodelling with resorption exceeding formation. This in turn leads to perforation of trabecular plates and loss of the underlying microstructure in trabecular bone, resulting in mechanical failure-fracture. Prevention and treatment of postmenopausal osteoporosis may be achieved by arresting bone resorption, or by stimulating bone formation. The former approach to date has been the most effective, using agents such as HRT.

HRT is effective in preventing bone loss and subsequent osteoporosis with its attendant fractures, even in the long term. Early prospective studies of oophorectomized women established that oestrogen could prevent bone loss and the development of osteoporosis in the long term (13). Long-term studies in women following natural menopause have supported the benefits on the skeleton suggested by retrospective population studies (14–16). Prospective randomized placebo-controlled studies confirm the reduction in fractures effected by oestrogen (17). Orally administered conjugated oestrogens 0.625 mg daily (18, 19), oestradiol 17β 1–2 mg daily (20), and oestrone sulphate 1.5 mg daily (21) have now been established as average bone-conserving doses. For transdermal oestradiol 17β, the usual bone-conserving dose is 50 μg daily (22) whilst for oestradiol 17β implants it is 50 mg (23) given every 6 months. HRT is equally effective in elderly women and in those who already have established osteoporis (24). Not only is there bone conservation, but also small increases in bone density can be achieved. Withdrawal of HRT leads to loss of bone, but only at the same rate as normal postmenopausal loss (25, 26). Thus any period of treatment with HRT buys time for the skeleton. Indeed, it has been estimated, for example, that just 5 years therapy would bring a reduction in the overall incidence of hip fracture of 50% (27).

Strategies for osteoporotic fracture prevention using HRT include both early and late intervention. Early intervention soon after the onset of menopause has the advantage of retaining the maximal amount of bone in the skeleton but requires long-term treatment which may be a potential drawback. Late intervention in women in their seventh decade or beyond has the advantage of a quick effect on fracture risk with short term treatment but has the drawbacks of less patient acceptability of HRT and of actual occurrence of fracture before treatment can take effect (28).

The World Health Organization guidelines for the definition of osteoporosis suggest a bone density measurement of more than 2.5 standard deviations (T −2.5) below that of average young adult sex-matched normals, irrespective of established fracture. Use of HRT should be considered in women with osteoporosis as demonstrated by this reduced bone density, although a better definition for those aged over 70 years might be a reduction in bone density of more than one standard deviation below the average for age- and sex-matched normals (Z −1.0). Obviously, women with radiographic or clinical osteoporosis should be treated without necessary resort to bone density measurement.

Osteoporosis treatment guidelines

Women with established risk for osteoporosis should be given HRT in an appropriate bone-conserving dose. The treatment should be continued for at least 5 years and preferably longer. Early intervention in young and prematurely postmenopausal women may require higher than average doses whereas late intervention in the elderly may be achieved with lower than average doses. A repeat bone density measurement after two years of therapy may be useful to determine whether the dose is effective in such cases.

Cardiovascular disease

The major cardiovascular diseases to affect women are coronary heart disease (CHD) and stroke. CHD is the major cause of death in women just as it is in men, and in many first world countries mortality from cardiovascular disease over all ages is actually slightly greater in females. Premenopausal females rarely get CHD, but loss of ovarian function leads to a clear increase in the disease (29−31). Since various adverse metabolic changes occur at the menopause, this suggests that the presence of ovarian hormones premenopausally protects against CHD; it therefore seems likely that HRT will do the same. Whilst as yet there have been no sufficiently large prospective randomised controlled trials of HRT and cardiovascular disease, the data from many epidemiological studies showing a protective effect are very solid. Postmenopausal oestrogen replacement results in a reduction in CHD of around 40−50% (32−34) and a reduction in stroke from between 30–50% (33–35). There are fewer data available for the use of oestrogen/progestogen HRT but those available suggest that progestogen addition does not negate the effect of oestrogen in terms of cardiovascular benefit (36, 37).

Benefits of oestrogen are also seen in women with established CHD, with an 87% reduction of CHD among oestrogen users in one recent study (38). An increase in survival over 10 years has also been reported with oestrogen use in postmenopausal women with CHD, with the greatest benefit seen in those with the most severe coronary atheroma (39). Thus there is really sufficient evidence to encourage the use of HRT in postmenopausal women with established risk of CHD.

The precise mechanisms by which sex steroids affect the cardiovascular system are still being investigated, but there are clearly both direct arterial effects and effects on metabolic risk factors for CHD.

Metabolic effects of HRT

HRT has effects on lipids and lipoproteins which are dependent on the type of oestrogen and progestogen used, and the route of administration. Oestrogens lower low density lipoprotein (LDL) cholesterol irrespective of type or route of administration (40), and this effect is not opposed by progestogens. Oral oestrogens will increase the concentrations of high density lipoprotein (HDL) cholesterol, particularly the important HDL_2 subfraction, whilst transdermal oestradiol has a somewhat lesser effect (40). However, this effect on HDL may be opposed by progestogens, particularly the more androgenic progestogens such as norgestrel (40). Transdermal oestradiol lowers triglycerides whereas conjugated equine oestrogens increase them (40). Oral oestradiol has relatively little effect on triglycerides, but androgenic progestogens reverse these oestrogen-induced rises. Overall, the effect of HRT on lipids and lipoproteins can be considered beneficial in terms of CHD. Insulin resistance is considered to be a pivotal metabolic disturbance leading to the development of CHD. Oestrogens tend to improve glucose and insulin metabolism by reducing insulin resistance although again this effect can be opposed by certain progestogens (41). In our studies, we have found that conjugated equine oestrogens, given together with cyclical norgestrel, are associated with deterioration of glucose tolerance and elevated insulin levels (42). The increase in insulin concentrations is due to an insufficient initial insulin response to the glucose challenge which results in a reduced glucose elimination rate at the start of the test and hence an overall elevation of glucose concentrations. This in turn stimulates an increased pancreatic insulin secretion and thus causes an overall increased insulin response. The addition of norgestrel to the conjugated equine oestrogens causes an increase in insulin resistance. With transdermal HRT, little effect on glucose and insulin metabolism is seen. In contrast, we have observed reduced insulin responses to an oral glucose challenge yet no deterioration in glucose tolerance when a C-21 progestogen, dydrogesterone, is given orally with oestradiol 17β, suggesting an improvement in insulin resistance (submitted for publication). It thus appears that oestradiol 17β has a beneficial effect on glucose and insulin metabolism whereas conjugated equine oestrogens may have some unwanted effects, and that the more androgenic progestogens result in an increase in insulin resistance which is avoided with the C-21 progestogens.

HRT may have other metabolic effects such as changes in body fat distribution and effects on coagulation and fibrinolysis which may contribute in part to its overall benefit to the cardiovascular system (43). Most of these metabolic effects would tend to reduce, or even reverse, the development of atheroma. The effects would therefore take some time to develop, but equally should persist for some time following cessation of therapy. In contrast, direct arterial effects of HRT should have fairly immediate actions but equally disappear rapidly on withdrawing treatment.

Direct arterial effects of HRT

Oestradiol exerts an inotropic effect in animals, causing systemic vasodilation and increased cardiac output (44). Studies of arterial waveform pulsatility index, an index inversely reflecting arterial compliance, in the carotid arteries of postmenopausal women have shown a steady increase in this parameter during the first few years following the monopause (45). This increase can be reversed by oestradiol 17β (45), and the effect is not abolished by progestogen addition (46). The acute administration of oestradiol 17β causes a reduction in myocardial ischaemia, as shown by an increase in time to 1 mm ST segment depression and in overall exercise time during the ECG exercise test, in postmenopausal women with established CHD (47). Postmenopausal oestrogen use also results in an overall decrease in blood pressure (35).

The actions of oestradiol on arteries is mediated through both endothelium-dependent and endothelium-independent mechanisms. Studies both in animals (48) and in women (49, 50) have shown that the endothelium-dependent vasodilator response to acetylcholine is improved by oestradiol administration.

However, oestradiol may also act through calcium-dependent mechanisms. In studies of isolated arterial rings, an increase in the calcium concentration of the medium resulted in contraction of the arterial rings but this effect was inhibited in a dose-dependent manner by the addition of oestradiol 17β (51). Oestradiol

17β also inhibits inward calcium currents and reduces intracellular free calcium in isolated cardiac myocytes (51). Continuous combined oestrogen and progestogen has been shown to reduce circulating angiotensin-I converting-enzyme (ACE) activity (52) and this may be another mechanism of vascular action. Finally, there is evidence that oestradiol inhibits vascular smooth muscle proliferation (53).

Cardiovascular treatment guidelines

HRT should be considered for use in women who have established risk for cardiovascular disease. These would include women who have had angina or a myocardial infarction, and those at high risk such as diabetics, hypertensives, hyperlipidaemics and smokers. There is some evidence that HRT has the same magnitude of benefit in terms of disease reduction in such patients (37). It is likely that other risk groups will be identified in the future. Little is known about the type of HRT necessary for the treatment of cardiovascular disease, but the choice of steroids and the route of administration will be governed by the particular metabolic features of the individual cases.

Concerns have been expressed about the use of progestogen addition, but as stated above the available data suggest that this does not impair the benefits of oestrogen. At present, there are insufficient data to know whether continuous combined HRT will have the same cardiovascular benefit as HRT with cyclical progestogen. It is also unknown whether tibolone will have such benefit. Doses necessary for cardiovascular protection have not been established but it would seem likely that doses at least equivalent to the bone-sparing doses of oestrogens should be used. Also the necessary duration of therapy is unknown, but in light of what is known about the mechanisms of action of HRT it would seem likely that the treatment would need to be given long-term if not indefinitely.

Conclusions

The benefits of HRT quite clearly outweigh any potential risks. It is the obvious treatment for the relief of menopausal symptoms due to oestrogen deficiency and is as effective as any other available therapy for the prevention and treatment of postmenopausal osteoporosis. It seems most likely that HRT will be effective in the prevention and treatment of cardiovascular disease, and its use should now be considered in women with established risk. HRT provides a unique health opportunity to aging women. Since it is not indicated in all women, unselected use of HRT is not appropriate, but it is clear that its more widespread use in the many women who need it must be a target for the future.

References

1. Persson I, Adami HO, Bergkvist L. Risk of endometrial cancer after treatment with oestrogens alone or in conjunction with progesterone: results of a prospective study. Br Med J 1988; 298: 147–151.
2. Cerin A, Heldaas K, Moeller B. Adverse endometrial effects of long-cycle estrogen and progestogen replacement therapy. N Engl J Med 1996; 334: 668–669.
3. Christiansen C, Riis BJ. Five years with continuous-combined oestrogen/progestogen therapy: effects on calcium metabolism, lipoproteins and bleeding patterns. Br J Obstet Gynaecol 1990; 97: 1087–1092.
4. Christiansen C, Riis BJ. 17β-estradiol and continuous norethisterone: a unique treatment for established osteoporosis in elderly women. J Clin Endocrinol Metab 1990; 71: 836–841.
5. Marsh MS, Crook D, Whitcroft SIJ, Worthington M, Whitehead MI, Stevenson JC. Effect of continuous combined estrogen and desogestrel hormone replacement therapy on serum lipids and lipoproteins. Obstet Gynecol 1994; 83: 19–23.
6. The Writing Group for the PEPI Trial. Effects of estrogen or estrogen/progestin regimens on heart disease risk factors in postmenopausal women. The Postmenopausal Estrogen/Progestin Interventions (PEPI) Trial. J Am Med Assoc 1995; 273: 199–208.
7. Rymer J, Chapman MG, Fogelman I. Effect of tibolone on postmenopausal bone loss. Osteoporosis Int 1994; 4: 314–319.
8. Rymer J, Crook D, Sidhu M, Chapman M, Stevenson JC. Effects of tibolone on serum concentrations of lipoprotein (a) in postmenopausal women. Acta Endocrinol 1993; 128: 259–262.
9. Steingold KA, Matt DW, DeZeigler D, Sealey JE, Fratkin M, Reznikov S. Comparison of transdermal to oral estradiol administration on hormonal and hepatic parameters in women with premature ovarian failure. J Clin Endocrinol Metab 1991; 73: 275–280.
10. Cardozo L. The role of oestrogens in urogynaecology. In: Birkauser M, Rozenbaum H, ed. Menopause. European Consensus Development Conference. Paris: Eska, 1996: 59–66.
11. Godsland IF, Rosano GMC, Proudler AJ, Collins P, Poole-Wilson P, Stevenson JC. Insulin resistance in postmenopausal women with syndrome X who do not respond to estrogen therapy. Circulation 1994; 90: 551–554.
12. Stevenson JC, Lees B, Devenport M, Cust MP, Ganger KF. Determinants of bone density in normal women: risk factors for future osteoporosis? Br Med J 1989; 298: 924–928.
13. Lindsay R, Hart DM, Aitken JM, MacDonald EB, Anderson JB, Clarke AC. Long-term prevention of postmenopausal osteoporosis by oestrogen. Lancet 1976; i: 1038–1041.
14. Hutchinson TA, Polansky SM, Feinstein AR. Postmenopausal oestrogens protect against fractures of the hip and distal radiums: a case controlled study. Lancet 1979; ii: 705–709.
15. Weiss NS, Ure BL, Ballard JH, Williams AR, Daling JR. Decreased risk of fractures of the hip and lower forearm with postmenopausal use of estrogen. N Engl J Med 1980; 303: 1195–1198.
16. Paganini-Hill A, Ross RK, Gerkins VR, Henderson BE, Arthur M, Mack TM. Menopausal oestrogen therapy and hip fractures. Ann Int Med 1981; 95: 28–31.
17. Lufkin EG, Wahner H, O'Fallon WM, et al. Treatment of postmenopausal osteoporosis with transdermal estradiol. Ann Intern Med 1992; 117: 1–9.
18. Lindsay R, Hart DM, Clark DM. The minimum effective dose of oestrogen for prevention of postmenopausal bone loss. Obstet Gynecol 1984; 63: 759–763.
19. Hillard TC, Whitcroft SIJ, Marsh MS, et al. Long-term effects of transdermal and oral hormone replacement therapy on postmenopausal bone loss. Osteoporosis Int 1994; 4: 341–348.
20. Christiansen C, Christensen MS, Larsen N-E, Transbol IB. Pathophysiological mechanisms of estrogen effect on bone metabolism. Dose-response relationships in early postmenopausal women. J Clin Endocrinol Metab 1982; 55: 1124–1130.
21. Harris ST, Genant HK, Baylink DJ, et al. The effects of estrone (Ogen) on spinal bone density of postmenopausal women. Arch Intern Med 1991; 151: 1980–1984.

22. Stevenson JC, Cust MP, Gangar KF, Hillard TC, Lees B, Whitehead MI. Effects of transdermal versus oral hormone replacement therapy on bone density in spine and proximal femur in postmenopausal women. Lancet 1990; 335: 265–269.
23. Studd J, Savvas M, Watson N, Garnett T,m Fogelman I, Cooper D. The relationship between plasma estradiol and the increase in bone density in post-menopausal women after treatment with subcutaneous hormone implants. Am J Obstet Gynecol 1990; 163: 1474–1479.
24. Lindsay R, Tohme JF. Estrogen treatment of patients with established postmenopausal osteoporosis. Obstet Gynecol 1990; 76: 290–295.
25. Christiansen C, Christensen MS, Transbol I. Bone mass in postmenopausal women after withdrawal of oestrogen/gestagen replacement therapy. Lancet 1981; 1: 459–461.
26. Stevenson JC, Kanis JA, Christansen C. Bone mass in women after withdrawal of oestrogen/ gestagen replacement therapy. Lancet 1992; 339: 370–371.
27. Stevenson JC. Post-menopausal bone loss and osteoporosis. In: Zichella L, Whitehead MI, van Keep PA, ed. The climacteric and beyond. Carnforth: Parthenon Publishing, 1988: 125–135.
28. Stevenson JC. Late prevention of hip fractures with hormone replacement therapy. Osteoporosis Int 1996; 6 suppl 3: in press.
29. Oliver MF, Boyd GS. Effect of bilateral ovariectomy on coronary artery disease and serum lipid levels. Lancet 1959; ii: 690–692.
30. Sznajderman M, Oliver MF. Spontaneous premature monopause, ischaemic heart disease and serum lipids. Lancet 1963; i: 962–964.
31. Gordon T, Kannel WB, Hjortland MC, McNamara PM. Menopause and coronary heart disease. The Framingham Study. Ann Intern Med 1978; 89: 157–161.
32. Hunt K, Vessey M, McPherson K. Mortality in a cohort of long-term users of hormone replacement therapy: an updated analysis. British Journal of Obstetrics and Gynaecology 1990; 97: 1080–1086.
33. Henderson B, Paganini-Hill A, Ross RK. Decreased mortality in users of estrogen replacement therapy. Arch Intern Med 1991; 151: 75–78.
34. Stampfer MJ, Grodstein F. Role of hormone replacement in cardiovascular disease. In: Lobo RA, ed. Treatment of the Postmenopausal Woman: Basic and Clinical Aspects. New York: Raven Press Ltd., 1994: 223–233.
35. Finucane FF, Madans JII, Bush TL, et al. Decreased risk of stroke among postmenopausal hormone users. Results from a national cohort. Arch Intern Med 1993; 153: 73–79.
36. Falkeborn M, Persson I, Adami H-O, et al. The risk of acute myocardial infarction after oestrogen and oestrogen-progestogen replacement. Br J Obstet Gynaecol 1992; 99: 821–828.
37. Psaty BM, Heckbert SR, Atkins D, et al. The risk of myocardial infarction associated with the combined use of estrogens and progestins in postmenopausal women. Arch Intern Med 1994; 1333–1339.
38. Hong MK, Romm PA, Reagan K, Green CE, Rackley CE. Effects of estrogen replacement therapy on serum lipid values and angiographically defined coronary artery disease in postmenopausal women. Am J Cardiol 1992; 69: 176–178.
39. Sullivan JM, Zwaag RV, Hughes JP, et al. Estrogen replacement therapy and coronary artery disease. Arch Intern Med 1990; 150: 2557–2562.
40. Crook D, Cust MP, Gangar KF, et al. Comparison of transdermal and oral estrogen/progestin hormone replacement therapy: effects on serum lipids and liporoteins. Am J Obstet Gynecol 1992; 166: 950–955.
41. Stevenson JC, Proudler AJ, Walton C, Godsland IF. HRT mechanisms of action: carbohydrates. Int J Fertil 1994; 39 (suppl 1): 50–55.
42. Godsland IF, Gangar KF, Walton C, et al. Insulin resistance, secretion, and elimination in postmenopausal women receiving oral or transdermal hormone replacement therapy. Metabolism 1993; 42: 846–853.

43. Stevenson JC. The metabolic and cardiovascular consequences of HRT. Br J Clin Pract 1995; 49: 87–90.
44. Magness RR, Rosenfeld CR. Local and systemic estradiol-17 beta: effects on uterine and systemic vasodilation. Am J Physiol 1989; 256: E536–E542.
45. Gangar KF, Vyas S, Whitehead M, Crook D, Meire H, Campbell S. Pulsatility index in internal carotid artery in relation to transdermal oestradiol and time since menopause. Lancet 1991; 338: 839–842.
46. Hillard TC, Bourne TH, Whitehead MI, Crayford TB, Collins WP, Campbell S. Differential effects of transdermal estradiol and sequential progestogens on impedance to flow within the uterine arteries of postmenopausal women. Fertility and Sterility 1992; 58: 959–963.
47. Rosano GMC, Sarrel PM, Poole-Wilson PA, Collins P. Beneficial effect of oestrogen on exercise-induced myocardial ischaemia in women with coronary artery disease. Lancet 1993; 342: 133–136.
48. Williams JK, Adams MR, Klopfenstein HS. Estrogen modulates responses of atherosclerotic coronary arteries. Circulation Res 1990; 81: 1680–1687.
49. Lieberman EH, Gerhard MD, Uehata A, et al. Estrogen improves endothelium-dependent, flow-mediated vasodilation in postmenopausal women. Ann Intern Med 1994; 121: 936–941.
50. Collins P, Rosano GMC, Sarrel PM, et al. 17β-estradiol attentuates acetylcholine-induced coronary arterial constriction in women but not men with coronary heart disease. Circulation 1995; 92: 24–30.
51. Jiang C, Poole-Wilson P, Sarrel P, Mochizuku S, Collins P. Effects of 17β-oestradiol on contraction, Ca^{2+} current and intracellular free Ca^{2+} in guinea-pig isolated cardiac myocytes. Br J Pharmacol 1992; 106: 739–745.
52. Proudler A, Ahmed A, Crook D, Fogelman I, Rymer J, Stevenson J. Hormone replacement therapy and serum angiotensin-converting-enzyme activity in postmenopausal women. Lancet 1995; 346: 89–90.
53. Mendelsohn ME, Karas RH. Estrogen and the blood vessel wall. Curr Opin Cardiol 1994; 9: 619–626.

5 The metabolic syndrome in postmenopausal women

Ian F. Godsland

The metabolic syndrome

Physiologic and metabolic risk factors for cardiovascular disease that have hitherto been considered in isolation are increasingly viewed in the context of syndromes of metabolic disturbance. This acknowledges the fact that adverse changes in one factor may induce adverse changes in a variety of other risk factors. In evaluating cardiovascular risk it is therefore useful to consider coordinated changes in risk factors, rather than attempt to isolate single, independent factors.

Recognition of risk factor interrelationships developed throughout the 1980s and culminated in Reaven's proposal that there was a distinct syndrome of metabolic disturbances – 'Syndrome X'; this syndrome had insulin resistance as its key aetiological factor (1). Confusion was engendered, however, since the term, Syndrome X, had previously been used to describe angina with an ischaemic exercise electrocardiogram and angiographically normal coronary arteries (2; see also Stevenson JC, chapter 4). The 'insulin resistance syndrome' is now the preferred designation, although even this obscures the fact that no formal clinical definition exists and manifestations of the syndrome may vary (3). The general concept of a 'metabolic syndrome' may be more realistic, and more useful, since it can allow for the identification of metabolic risk profiles characteristic of specific conditions, such as non-insulin-dependent diabetes mellitus, hypertension, familial combined hyperlipidaemia, visceral obesity, or, as will be described below, the postmenopausal state.

Risk factors that have been found to exhibit significant mechanistic or statistical inter-relationships in the context of the metabolic syndrome include: insulin resistance, impaired glucose tolerance, hyperinsulinaemia, elevated triglyceride and reduced high density lipoprotein (HDL) concentrations, increased visceral adiposity and blood pressure, elevated uric acid concentrations, increased plasminogen activator inhibitor-1 (PAI-1) activity, an impaired vasodilatory response to insulin, impaired postprandial triglyceride clearance, and increased proportion of the small dense low density lipoprotein (LDL) subfraction (4).

A number of mechanisms have been identified which would be expected to contribute to these 'core' disturbances of the metabolic syndrome. Providing pancreatic insulin responsiveness to glucose is normal, hyperinsulinaemia is an inevitable consequence of insulin resistance since insulin levels must rise to maintain normoglycaemia in the face of resistance to insulin action. Although fasting glucose levels are not affected, glucose concentrations following a glucose load may fall more slowly in states of insulin resistance since, although the augmented insulin response may be sufficient to normalise blood glucose levels, it may not fully compensate for raised post-load glucose levels (5). A number of enzymes of lipid and lipoprotein metabolism are insulin sensitive (6). Adipose tissue hormone sensitive lipase is strongly suppressed by insulin, so insulin resistance with respect to this enzyme will result in impaired suppression of lipolysis by insulin, increased supply of non-esterified fatty acids to the liver and increased triglyceride synthesis. Lipoprotein lipase (LPL) activity is stimulated by insulin (7), so insulin resistance with respect to this enzyme will result in decreased LPL activity, decreased triglyceride clearance from the circulation and increased postprandial lipaemia. Hepatic triglyceride lipase participates in the conversion of the important HDL_2 subfraction to the HDL_3 subfraction, low levels of which are seen in states of increased vascular disease risk. Hepatic lipase activity may be stimulated by insulin (8), so the increased hepatic insulinisation that accompanies insulin resistance may diminish HDL_2 levels (9). Insulin stimulates catecholamine release and renal sodium reabsorption, both of which would be expected to increase blood pressure (10). Normally these effects may be counteracted by insulin-stimulated vasodilation, but in states of insulin resistance this vasodilation is impaired, thus accounting for the associations reported between insulin resistance, hyperinsulinaemia and increased blood pressure (11). The increased triglyceride synthesis and decreased triglyceride elimination associated with insulin resistance have effects on other aspects of lipoprotein metabolism, leading to decreased levels of HDL, and increased proportions of atherogenic small, dense LDL (12). Also linked with increased non-esterified fatty acid flux and increased triglyceride synthesis is an increased proportion of central, visceral or android adipose tissue, which is particularly sensitive to lipolytic hormones and thus has a high intrinsic rate of lipolysis (13). Finally, links with the coagulation and haemostatic systems have been distinguished; in particular, synthesis of PAI-1 is stimulated by insulin (14).

Hypercholesterolemia has not previously been considered as a component of any metabolic syndrome. However there are points of convergence: insulin resistance may be present in certain states of hypercholesterolemia (15) and elevated cholesterol levels induce endothelial dysfunction which, because insulin action depends on endothelial transcytosis (16), would be expected to contribute to insulin resistance. Moreover, raised cholesterol may contribute to atherogenesis via oxidation of small, dense LDL. Lipoprotein (a), elevated levels of which have been linked with cardiovascular disease, appears to be independent of the classic metabolic syndrome, but may be linked to insulin secretion (17). Serum angiotensin converting enzyme (ACE) activity shows no interrelationship with any of the core components of the metabolic syndrome (18, 19).

Menopause and the metabolic syndrome

In considering the metabolic syndrome in postmenopausal women, several critical underlying considerations must be born in mind. Firstly, there will be correlated disturbances which have as their common aetiological factor the decline in oestrogen levels that accompanies the menopause. These disturbances will then themselves have effects which may augment the effects of the menopause. The second consideration is that there will be two components to the emergence of risk factor disturbances after the menopause; disturbances which appear during the climacteric, and disturbances which develop progressively with increasing time since menopause.

In comparison with premenopausal women, or in analyses in which risk factor variation with increasing menopausal rather than chronological age has been distinguished, the following characteristics have been linked with the menopause and the postmenopausal state:

- increase in serum total and LDL cholesterol (20)
- increased triglycerides (21)
- decreased triglyceride elimination (22)
- decreased HDL (20)
- increased small dense LDL (23)
- increased lipoprotein (a)(24)
- increased insulin resistance (25, 26)
- decreased insulin elimination (27)
- decrease in pancreatic insulin secretion (27)
- impaired vascular function (28)
- increased visceral adiposity (29)
- increased uric acid concentrations (Wynn Institute – unpublished data)
- increased fibrinogen (30)
- increased factor VII (31)
- increased blood pressure (32)

These changes are described in detail below, with particular reference to the circumstantial evidence for their importance, and the mechanisms responsible, that comes from studies of oestrogen replacement and experimental studies of the effects of estrogens in vitro.

Effects of the menopause on lipid and lipoprotein metabolism

Oestrogens upregulate the hepatic LDL receptor and accelerate receptor-mediated LDL catabolism (33). They may also stimulate hepatic excretion of cholesterol in the bile (34). Therefore, loss of oestrogens at the menopause would be expected to be accompanied by a rise on total and LDL cholesterol levels. In fact, a rise in LDL cholesterol concentrations of up to 25% has been reported (21).

The effects of oestrogens on triglyceride metabolism are confounded by the stimulation of hepatic triglyceride synthesis and increased production of large triglyceride-rich very low density lipoprotein (VLDL) that has been seen consistently with orally administered oestrogens (33). It is possible that this is a specific effect of the high oestrogen concentrations to which the liver is exposed when oestrogen is administered by the oral root – the so-called 'hepatic first pass effect'. Transdermally adminstered oestradiol appears to have considerably less effect on triglyceride levels (33) and may even cause a reduction (35). This could be associated with the increased postprandial triglyceride elimination that has been reported in response to oestradiol administration (36). The increased triglyceride levels that have been consistently seen in association with menopause, both natural and surgical, might then be accounted for by decreased triglyceride elimination after the menopause, and there is some evidence for this (22). An increase in the proportion of small, dense LDL is consistently seen in association with increased triglyceride levels, probably because of altered very low density lipoprotein (VLDL) and LDL metabolism when these lipoprotein particles are triglyceride-enriched (23). Postmenopausal women appear to have raised levels of small, dense LDL, but, paradoxically, oestrogens appear to increase the proportion of small, dense LDL (37). However, the oestrogens that have been evaluated so far, with respect to effects on LDL subfractions, tend to increase triglyceride levels. Physiological replacement of oestrogen might not have such an effect on the LDL subfractions.

Oestrogens stimulate the synthesis of the principal apoprotein of HDL, apo AI (38), and suppress hepatic triglyceride lipase activity (39). Loss of these effects following the menopause would be expected to result in a decline in HDL levels, particularly in the HDL_2 subfraction, as has been observed (20). Menopause is associated with a rise in Lp(a) levels and, in accord with this, oestrogens appear to lower Lp(a) levels (40).

Effects of the menopause on insulin and glucose metabolism

Menopause as such does not appear to affect fasting or glucose tolerance test glucose and insulin levels, but there do appear to underlying changes and progressive changes following the menopause (26). Menopause is associated with a decline in glucose-stimulated insulin secretion (27). This accords with much early work on animal models for diabetes in which oestrogens were found to have a protective effect (41), and later work demonstrating increased insulin secretion from panceatic islets isolated from oestrogen-treated animals (42). In humans, the menopausal decline in insulin secretion appears to be compensated by a reduction in peripheral insulin elimination, so, although reduced in quantity, insulin remains in the circulation significantly longer.

With regard to insulin resistance, experimental studies have shown an improvement in the metabolic response to insulin in tissues isolated from oestrogen-treated animals (43) and there is some evidence for this from studies in humans. Progesterone has the opposite effect, so the decline in both hormones at the menopause might be expected to result in no overall effect on insulin resistance. This has been observed (27), but it is also apparent that, following the menopause, there is a progressive increase in insulin resistance, and this relates to time since menopause rather than chronological age (25).

Effects of the menopause on haemostasis

Factor VII and fibrinogen, both independent predictors of coronary heart disease, appear to be raised in postmenopausal compared with premenopausal women (30, 31). The antifibrinolytic factor PAI-1 may also be increased, since levels of PAI-1 rise with age after the menopause, in contrast to the fall with age that is seen in premenopausal women (44). There is some evidence that there may be compensatory increases in the antithrombotic and antifibrinolytic factors antithrombin-III and plasminogen after the menopause (45).

Effects of the menopause on body fat distribution, vascular function and blood pressure

An increased proportion of centrally located (visceral or android) body fat is a strong correlate of adverse changes in blood pressure and in a range of metabolic risk factors for cardiovascular disease (46). It is also an independent predictor of coronary heart disease (47). Postmenopausal women have an increased proportion of central body fat compared with premenopausal women (29), and there is some evidence for redistribution to a more peripheral pattern in response to oestrogen (48).

Some deterioration in vascular function after the menopause has been suggested by the report of a significant increase in the internal carotid artery pulsatility index with increasing time since menopause (28). Moreover, this is reversed by oestrogen replacement (26). Effects of the menopause on serum ACE activity do not appear to have been investigated, but a decline in ACE activity in response to oestrogen replacement has been observed in postmenopausal women, suggesting that there might indeed be some increase in ACE activity at or after the menopause (49). Some increase in blood pressure after the menopause, beyond an age-related increase, might be expected to accompany the changes in insulin resistance, body fat distribution and pulsatility index in postmenopausal women. There is evidence for an overall increase in blood pressure in postmenopausal women (32), and for an oestrogen-induced reduction in blood pressure (50), but a number of studies have also reported no change.

Risk factor interrelationships after the menopause

A broad range of risk factors for cardiovascular disease are favourably affected by oestrogens, the decline in oestrogen concentrations after the menopause is associated with a number of adverse changes in risk factor levels that are consistent with this, and oestrogen replacement after the menopause can reverse these changes. It, therefore, seems reasonable to propose a menopausal syndrome of metabolic disturbances which have as their common aetiological factor oestrogen deficiency. These disturbances may themselves be interrelated. For example, the progressive decline in insulin sensitivity and the progressive increase in pulsatility index after the menopause recall the impaired vasodilation in response to insulin in insulin resistant states (11). Such states include obesity, which provides a link with the increased central fat seen after the menopause. Relationships between insulin and the haemostatic system may be more extensive than hitherto supposed. We have recently observed significant positive correlations between intravenous glucose tolerance test insulin response and fibrinogen, factor VII and factor X levels, in addition to the well-established association between insulin and PAI-1 (Wynn Institute – unpublished data).

Conclusions

It has long been accepted that postmenopausal women are at an appreciably increased risk of cardiovascular disease compared with their premenopausal counterparts, and epidemiological studies suggest that oestrogen replacement in postmenopausal women may reduce cardiovascular disease incidence by up to 50%. Changes in risk factors for cardiovascular disease after the menopause have been linked with oestrogen deficiency and are consistent with the increased risk in postmenopausal women. Moreover, their amelioration by oestrogen replacement is consistent with the protective effect of oestrogens. The range of adverse changes in risk factors in response to oestrogen deficiency – and the resemblance of many of these changes to those seen in previously defined metabolic syndromes – justifies adoption of the concept of a distinct menopausal metabolic syndrome. Any long-term therapy to be prescribed to postmenopausal women should not exacerbate this syndrome.

References

1. Reaven G. Banting Lecture 1988: role of insulin resistance in human disease. Diabetes 1988; 37: 1595–1607.
2. Kemp HG. Left ventricular function in patients with the anginal syndrome and normal coronary arteriograms. Am J Cardiol 1973; 32: 375–376.
3. Godsland IF, Stevenson JC. Insulin resistance: syndrome or tendency. Lancet 1995; 346: 100–103.
4. Després J-P, Marette A. Relation of components of insulin resistance syndrome to coronary disease risk. Curr Opin Lipidol 1994; 5: 274–289.
5. Hollenbeck C, Reaven GM. Variations in insulin-stimulated glucose uptake in healthy individuals with normal glucose tolerance. J Clin Endocrinol Metab 1987; 64: 1169–1173.
6. Frayn K. Insulin resistance and lipid metabolism. Curr Opin Lipidol 1993; 4: 197–204.
7. Sadur C, Eckel R. Insulin stimulation of adipose tissue lipoprotein lipase. J Clin Invest 1982; 69: 1119–1125.
8. Baynes C, Henderson AD, Richmond W, Johnston DG, Elkeles RS. The response of hepatic lipase and serum lipoproteins to acute hyperinsulinaemia in type 2 diabetes. Eur J Clin Invest 1992; 22: 341–346.
9. Godsland IF, Crook D, Walton C, Wynn V, Oliver MF. Influence of insulin resistance, secretion, and clearance on serum cholesterol, triglycerides, lipoprotein cholesterol, and blood pressure in healthy men. Arteriosclerosis and Thrombosis 1992; 12: 1030–1035.
10. Morris AD, Petrie JR, Connell JMC. Insulin and hypertension. J Hypertens 1994; 12: 633–642.
11. Baron AD. Hemodynamic actions of insulin. Am J Physiol 1994; 267: E187–E202.
12. Krauss R. The tangled web of coronary risk factors. Am J Med 1991; 90 (suppl 2A): 36–41.
13. Björntorp P. Metabolic implications of body fat distribution. Diabetes Care 1991; 14: 1132–1143.
14. Juhan-Vague I, Alessi M, Vague P. Increased plasminogen activator inhibitor 1 levels: A possible link between insulin resistance and atherothrombosis. Diabetologia 1991; 34: 457–462.
15. Castro Cabezas M, Bruin TWA, de Walk HW, Shoulders CC, Jansen H, Erkelens DW. Impaired fatty acid metabolism in familial combined hyperlipidemia: a mechanism associating apolipoprotein B overproduction and insulin resistance. J Clin Invest 1993; 92: 160–168.
16. Vilaró S, Palacín M, Pilch P, Testar X, Zorzano A. Expression of an insulin-regulatable glucose carrier in muscle and fat endothelial cells. Nature 1989; 342: 798–800.
17. Sidhu M, Crook D, Godsland I, Walton C, Wynn V, Oliver M. Inverse relationship between serum Lp(a) levels and first-phase insulin secretion. Diabetes 1992; 41: 1341–1345.
18. Proudler AJ, Crook D, Godsland IF, Collins P, Rosano GMC, Stevenson JC. Serum angiotensin 1-converting enzyme (ACE) activity in women with cardiological syndrome X: relation with blood pressure, and lipid and carbohydrate metabolic risk markers for coronary heart disease. J Clin Endocrinol Metab 1995; 86: 696–699.
19. Panahloo A, Andrès C, Mohamed-Ali V, Gould MM, Talmud P, Humphries SE, Yudkin JS. The insertion allele of the ACE gene I/D polymorphism. Circulation 1995; 92: 3390–3393.
20. Stevenson J, Crook D, Godsland I. Influence of age and menopause on serum lipids and lipoproteins in healthy women. Atherosclerosis 1993; 98: 83–90.
21. Jensen J, Nilas L, Christiansen C. Influence of menopause on serum lipids and lipoproteins. Maturitas 1990; 12: 321–331.
22. Tollin C, Ericsson M, Johnson O, Backman C. Clearance of triglycerides from the circulation and its relationship to serum lipoproteins: influence of age and sex. Scan J Clin Lab Invest 1985; 45: 679–684.
23. Selby JV, Austin MA, Newman B, Zhang D, Quesenberry CP, Mayer EJ, Krauss RM. LDL subclass phenotypes and the insulin resistance syndrome in women. Circulation 1993; 88: 381–387.

24. Meilahan EN, Kuller LH, Matthews KA, Stein EA. Lp(a) concentrations among pre- and post-menopausal women over time: the Healthy Women Study. Circulation 1991; 84 (sup II): 546 (abstract).
25. Proudler A, Felton C, Stevenson J. Ageing and the response of plasma insulin, glucose and C-peptide concentrations to intravenous glucose in postmenopausal women. Clin Sci 1992; 83: 489–494.
26. Godsland IF, Walton C, Stevenson JC. Impact of menopause on metabolism. In: Diamond MP, Naftolin F, eds. Metabolism in the Female Life Cycle. Ares Serono Symposia: Rome 1993; 171–189.
27. Walton C, Godsland IF, Proudler A, Wynn V, Stevenson J. The effects of the menopause on insulin sensitivity, secretion and elimination in nonobese, healthy women Eur J Clin Invest 1993; 23: 466–473
28. Gangar KF, Vyas S, Whitehead M, Crook D, Meire H, Campbell S. Pulsatility index in internal carotid artery in relation to transdermal oestradiol and time since menopause. Lancet 1991; 338: 839–842.
29. Ley C, Lees B, Stevenson J. Sex- and menopause-associated changes in body fat distribution. Am J Clin Nutr 1992; 55: 950–954.
30. Balleisen L, Bailey J, Epping P-H, Schulte H, van de Loo J. Epidemiological study on factor VII, factor VIII and fibrinogen in an industrial population. I Baseline data on the relation of age, gender, body weight, smoking, alcohol, pill use and menopause. Thromb Haemostasis 1985; 54: 475–479.
31. Scarabin P-Y, Bonithon-Kopp C, Malmejac BL, Guize L. Factor VII activation and menopausal status. Thromb Res 1990; 57: 227–234.
32. Staessen J, Bulpitt CJ, Fagard R, Lijnen P, Amery A. The influence of menopause on blood pressure. J Hum Hypertens 1989; 3: 427–433.
33. Walsh BW, Schiff I, Rosner B, Greenberg L, Ravnikar V, Sacks FM. Effects of postmenopausal estrogen replacement on the concentrations and metabolism of plasma lipoproteins. N Engl J Med 1991; 325: 1196–1204.
34. Kushwaha RS, Born KM. Effect of oestrogen and progesterone on the hepatic cholesterol 7 alpha-hydroxylase activity in ovariectomised baboons. Biochem Biophys Acta 1991; 1084: 300–302.
35. Crook D, Cust M, Gangar K, Worthington M, Hillard T, Stevenson J, Whitehead M, Wynn V. Comparison of transdermal and oral estrogen-progestin replacement therapy: effects on serum lipids and lipoproteins. Am J Obstet Gynecol 1992; 166: 950–955.
36. Westerveld HT, Kock LAW, van Rijn JM, Erkelens DW, de Bruin TWA. 17β-estradiol improves postprandial lipid metabolism in postmenopausal women. J Clin Endocrinol Metab 1995; 80: 249–253.
37. Campos H, Sacks FM, Walsh BW, Schiff I, O'Hanesian MA, Krauss RM. Differential effects of estrogen on low-density lipoprotein subclasses in healthy postmenopausal women. Metabolism 1993; 42: 1153–1158.
38. Schaefer E, Foster D, Zech L, Lindgren F, Brewer Jr H, Levy R. The effects of estrogen administration on plasma lipoprotein metabolism in premenopausal females. J Clin Endocrinol Metab 1983; 57: 262–267.
39. Tikkanen M, Nikkilä E, Kuusi T, Sipinen S. High density lipoprotein-2 and hepatic lipase: Reciprocal changes produced by estrogen and norgestrel. J Clin Endocrinol Metab 1982; 54: 1113–1117.
40. Sacks FM, McPherson R, Walsh B. Effect of postmenopausal estrogen replacement on plasma Lp(a) lipoprotein concentrations. Arch Intern Med 1994; 154: 1106–1110.
41. Rodriguez R. Influence of oestrogens and androgens on the production and prevention of diabetes. In: Leibel B, Wrenshall G, eds. On the nature and treatment of diabetes. Excerpta Medica: New York 1965; 288–307.

42. Costrini N, Kalkhoff R. Relative effects of pregnancy, estradiol and progesterone on plasma insulin and pancreatic islet insulin secretion. J Clin Invest 1971; 50: 992–999.
43. Rushakoff R, Kalkhoff R. Effects of pregnancy and sex steroid administration on skeletal muscle metabolism in the rat. Diabetes 1981; 30: 545–550.
44. Winkler UH. Menopause, hormone replacement therapy and cardiovascular disease: a review of haemostaseological findings. Fibrinolysis 1992; 6 (suppl 3): 5–10.
45. Meade TW, Dyer S, Howarth DJ, Imeson JD, Stirling Y. Antithrombin III and procoagulant activity: sex differences and effects of the menopause. Br J Haemtol 1990; 74: 77–81.
46. Ostlund Jr R, Staten M, Kohrt W, Schultz J, Malley M. The ratio of waist-to-hip circumference, plasma insulin level, and glucose intolerance as independent predictors of the HDL_2 cholesterol level in older adults. N Engl J Med 1990; 322: 229–234.
47. Lapidus I, Bengtsson C, Larsson B, Pennert K, Rybo F, Sjöström I. Distribution of adipose tissue and risk of cardiovascular disease and death: a 12 year follow up of participants in the population study of women in Gothenburg, Sweden. Br Med J 1984; 289: 1257–1261.
48. Haarbo J, Marslew U, Gotfredsen A, Christiansen C. Postmenopausal hormone replacement therapy prevents central distribution of body fat after menopause. Metabolism 1991; 40: 1323–1326.
49. Proudler AJ, Ahmed AIH, Crook D, Fogelman I, Rymer JM, Stevenson JC. Hormone replacement therapy and serum angiotensin converting enzyme (ACE) activity in postmenopausal women: a possible cardioprotective mechanism. Lancet 1995; 346: 89–90.
50. Barrett-Connor E, Brown WV. Heart disease risk factors and hormone use in postmenopausal women. JAMA 1979; 241: 2167–2169.

6 The clinical development of the new ACE-inhibitor moexipril

Michael Stimpel and Brigitte Koch

Introduction

As a class, angiotensin converting-enzyme inhibitors (ACE) have shown to be efficacious in the treatment of hypertension and congestive heart failure (1, 2). Since they have an excellent safety and tolerance profile (3, 4), they figure prominently in the therapy of these disorders.

This brief review summarizes the presently available clinical data on moexipril, a new, long-acting ACE-inhibitor, which has been developed for the once-a-day treatment of primary hypertension. At present (7/1996), moexipril is approved for this indication in the USA and in different European countries.

Pharmacological characteristics

Moexipril is a prodrug, which, following oral administration, is hydrolysed in vivo to its active carboxylic metabolite, moexiprilat, a nonsulfhydryl ACE-inhibitor. – As reported for other ACE-inhibitors e. g. benazepril (37%), fosinopril (32%), and lisinopril (30%) (5–7), an incomplete absorption has also been found for moexipril, with a low bioavailability of unchanged moexipril of about 20% (data on file, Schwarz Pharma). Twenty-four hours after oral intake of a single dose of moexipril, the activity of the angiotensin converting enzyme is still inhibited by 80% (8). Moexipril and moexiprilat are excreted by both the kidney and the liver. While most other ACE inhibitors are primarily excreted by the kidney, an extensive biliary excretion has also been reported for fosinopril (9) and ramipril (10).

The elemination half-life is approximately 10 hours and does not change with increasing doses (data on file, Schwarz Pharma). However, half-life is increasing with decreasing kidney function, and therefore it is recommended to adapt the dosage of moexipril in patients with a creatinine clearance of < 40 ml/min. More detailed reports on the pharmacokinetic and pharmacologic properties of moexipril have been published recently (11, 12).

Clinical use

All therapeutic trials of moexipril have involved either mild to moderate or moderate to severe primary hypertension. So far, no data are available on its therapeutic efficacy in indications such as congestive heart failure, for which ACE inhibitors as a class have generally been claimed to be effective.

Therapeutic efficacy

Mild to moderate hypertension

In clinical trials investigating the effect of moexipril in mild to moderate hypertension, patients underwent a 2- to 4-week placebo run-in period during which all antihypertensive medication was discontinued. At the end of this interval patients who remained hypertensive (diastolic blood pressure ≥ 95 mmHg) entered the treatment phase of the study, which typically lasted 8 to 12 weeks. In some trials the dosage of moexipril (and that of the comparator agent where applicable) was titrated to response at intervals of 4 weeks; also, in some other studies a diuretic was added to the regimen if blood pressure remained elevated despite increasing the dosage of the ACE-inhibitor. The assessment of the efficacy of moexipril was based on changes of primary efficacy parameters.

In most studies, sitting diastolic blood pressure (SDBP) 22–26 hours after the previous dose was used as the primary efficacy parameter. Patients responding to treatment were defined as those with a SDBP of < 90 mmHg or a reduction in SDBP of > 10 mmHg.

Placebo-controlled studies

All of the placebo-controlled studies of moexipril have been performed as multicentre studies in the USA and different European countries (13–20). Peak reduction of blood pressure by 7.5 mg or 15 mg moexipril is generally achieved in hypertensive patients within three to six hours. The maximum effect of a given once-daily dosage regimen of moexipril was reached after four weeks administration although most of the effect was evident already after two weeks (13).

Data from ambulatory blood pressure measurements, trough/peak ratios, and a comparison from dose-response studies using twice-daily and once-daily dosing schedules indicate that a once-daily schedule with dosages of 7.5 mg, 15 mg and 30 mg moexipril provides sufficient control of blood pressure over a 24-hour period in the majority of patients with mild to moderate hypertension (13, 17, 18). The dose-response relationship of once-daily doses of moexipril has been investigated in some clinical multidose studies. Dosages of 7.5 mg to 30 mg moexipril lowered SDBP and sitting systolic blood pressure (SSBP) at trough by 3 to 6 mmHg and to

4 to 11 mmHg, more than placebo, respectively. Results on the lowest tested dose, 3.75 mg, were contradictory showing a significant antihypertensive effect in one study (18) and no difference from placebo in another (13).

Comparative studies

In comparison with other standard antihypertensive agents such as hydrochlorothiazide 25 mg once daily (13, 14), captopril 25 to 50 mg twice daily (21) (Fig. 6.1) and verapamil SR 120–240 mg once daily (22) moexipril in dosages of 7.5 mg and 15 mg once daily has proved to be about equally efficacious in lowering blood pressure in patients with mild to moderate hypertension. In elderly patients (>65 years), the antihypertensive effect of 15 mg moexipril once daily was comparable with that of 25 mg HCTZ once daily (14).

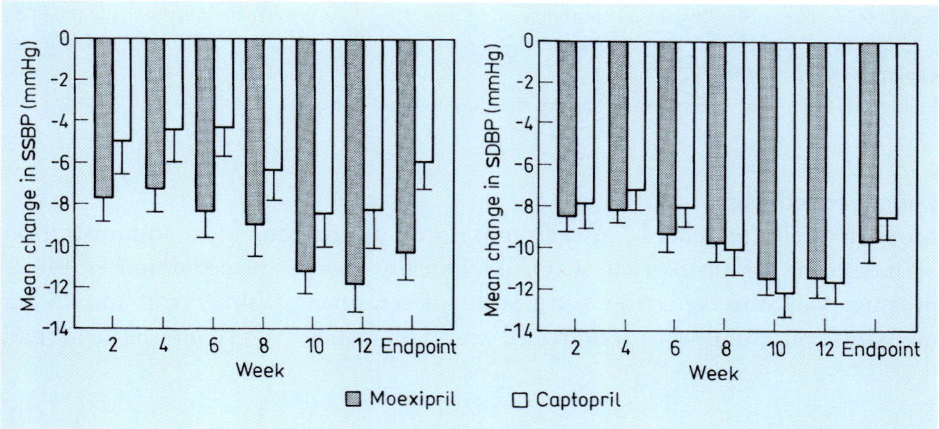

Figure 6.1: Effect of moexipril once-daily (7.5–15 mg/d) versus captopril twice-daily (25–50 mg/d) on systolic (SSBP; left side) and diastolic blood pressure (SDBP; right side) in patients (n = 159) with mild to moderate hypertension.

Combination studies

Since it is known that a stimulated RAS increases the antihypertensive efficacy of ACE inhibitors (23), moexipril was thoroughly investigated in combination with HCTZ. Two studies with a multifactorial design demonstrated that combinations of moexipril 3.75 mg to 30 mg with HCTZ 3.125 mg to 50 mg were more effective in lowering blood pressure than the individual components alone (18, 24). Even the extremely low-dosed combination of moexipril 3.75 mg/HCTZ 6.125 mg turned out to be statistically significantly more effective than placebo; this result was confirmed by another placebo-controlled study (Fig. 6.2), in which 200 patients with mild to moderate hypertension were enrolled (25).

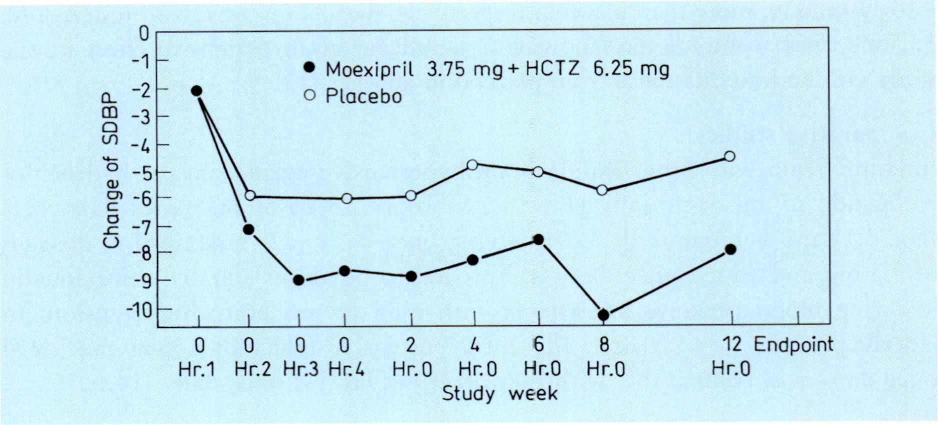

Figure 6.2: Effect of a low-dosed combination of moexipril 3.75 mg/hydrochlorothiazide (HCTZ) 6.25 mg versus placebo on sitting diastolic blood pressure (SDBP) in patients with mild to moderate hypertension (n = 200)[1].

[1] Last HF. 0 (trough) measurement during the double-blind period.

Long-term efficacy

More than 500 patients have been monitored during long-term administration of moexipril for up to two years. A clinically significant reduction of blood pressure was observed after six months of treatment with 7.5 mg and 15 mg moexipril once-daily in a controlled study, in which half of the patients had

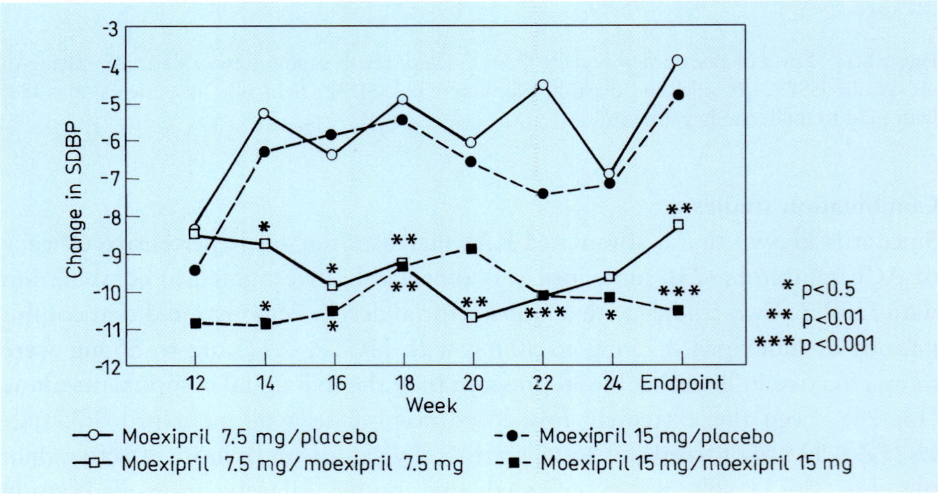

Figure 6.3: Changes in sitting diastolic blood pressure (SDBP) in patients after withdrawal of moexipril or in patients continuing on moexipril (randomized patients: n = 223).

been withdrawn from active treatment after three months and had subsequently been treated with placebo for the rest of the study. While blood pressure increased to baseline values two weeks after withdrawal, no tolerance developed under active treatment till the end of the study (16) (Fig. 6.3). In three open, uncontrolled studies hypertensive patients were treated for one year (data on file, Schwarz Pharma) or for two years (26, 27) with moexipril alone or in combination with HCTZ. The starting dose in all studies was 7.5 mg moexipril; in case of insufficient response the dosage could be increased to 15 mg (27) or 30 mg (26). Patients who did not respond to a once-daily monotherapy additionally received HCTZ 12.5 mg or 25 mg. The patients enrolled into these studies were taken from those who had previousely participated in placebo-controlled studies and had diastolic blood pressures of ≥95 mmHg to ≤114 mmHg at the end of the 4-week run-in period of these studies. In one of these studies only elderly patients (≥65 years of age) were investigated (27). After 12 (data on file, Schwarz Pharma; 26, 27) and 24 (26, 27) months moexipril alone and in combination with HCTZ decreased the SDBP statistically and clinically significant as compared with the pretreatment values.

The responder rates to moexipril monotherapy in these long-term studies were 67%, 72%, and 71% (data on file, Schwarz Pharma; 26, 27). Under all regimens, reductions of SDBP were maintained without any need for significant dose changes.

Moderate to severe hypertension

Three controlled studies were outlined to determine the efficacy of moexipril as add-on therapy to preexisting antihypertensive treatment in moderate to severe hypertension. After a 4-week treatment with either 25 mg HCTZ administered once-daily (19, 28) or 20 mg sustained release nifedipine twice-daily (20) patients were included into the study, if they had still elevated diastolic blood pressures of ≥95 mmHg to ≤114 mmHg. Subsequently, combined treatments of nifedipine/moexipril (20) as well as HCTZ/moexipril (19, 28) were significantly more effective in lowering blood pressure than nifedipine/placebo and HCTZ/placebo, respectively. In another study, the add-on effect of moexipril was compared to that of verapamil SR in patients with moderate to severe hypertension pretreated for 4 weeks with 25 mg HCTZ (28). In patients, who did not respond to the initial once-daily dosages of moexipril 7.5 mg (+HCTZ 25 mg) or verapamil SR 180 mg (+HCTZ 25 mg) after 4 weeks, the dosages were increased to 15 mg once-daily and 240 mg once-daily, respectively. The decrease in diastolic blood pressure, as compared to the pretreatment values, was −10.0 mmHg in the moexipril group and −7.5 mmHg in the verapamil group at the end of the first 4-week period, and −10.7 mmHg and −11.2 mmHg, respectively, at the end of the study.

In summary, all three studies showed an additional antihypertensive effect of moexipril in patients whose blood pressure was not sufficiently controlled by antihypertensive monotherapy. Under these conditions, moexipril was as effective as verapamil SR and proved to be statistically and clinically significantly more effective than placebo.

Efficacy in special populations

The effectiveness of moexipril in elderly and younger patients, in black and non-black races and in males and females was analysed retrospectively using pooled data from different controlled clinical studies (data on file, Schwarz Pharma). Except for one study showing a slightly favourable effect for women (25), no significant difference in antihypertensive efficacy of moexipril could be detected between male and female patients with hypertension. – Mean reductions in diastolic blood pressure for black hypertensives were approximately 2 mmHg to 3 mmHg less than corresponding reductions for non-black patients. With the caveat that only a restricted number of black hypertensives were treated placebo-controlled, moexipril appears to be slightly less effective in these patients. Similar observations have been made with beta-blockers and other ACE-inhibitors (29). The efficacy of moexipril in patients above or below 65 years of age did not differ significantly. At endpoint, the decrease of diastolic blood pressure was −1.2 mmHg more in the elderly. In a controlled comparative study, moexipril proved to be as efficacious as HCTZ in elderly patients after 12 weeks of treatment (14). A sustained antihypertensive effect for 2 years was demonstrated in 120 patients (≥65 years) receiving moexipril alone or in combination with HCTZ (27). In 20 patients with mild to moderate hypertension and concomitant renal insufficiency an average decrease in SDBP of −13.0 mmHg was observed after a maximal treatment period of 10 weeks (data on file, Schwarz Pharma).

Tolerability

The safety profile of moexipril does not essentially differ from that reported for other ACE-inhibitors (3, 4). Experience on safety with moexipril is based on data from clinical trials performed in approximately 3,400 hypertensive patients and 400 healthy volunteers. More than 500 of these patients were treated with moexipril for 1 to 2 years (26, 27; data on file, Schwarz Pharma).

The overall incidence of reported adverse events was similar in patients treated with moexipril (53%) to that reported in patients treated with placebo (47%). Only 20% of those adverse events seen under treatment with moexipril were classified as possibly or probably drug-related (Table 6.1). Reported adverse events were usually mild and transient, and there were no differences in adverse reaction rates related to gender, race, age, duration of therapy, or total daily

Table 6.1: Percentage of patients with adverse events (AE), possibly or probably drug related listed according to frequency*.

Adverse events	Moexipril n = 1355	Moexipril/ HCTZ n = 604	HCTZ n = 327	Placebo n = 417
all AEs	20	21	19	11
Headache	4	2	2	3
Cough	4	4	1	1
Dizziness	3	3	2	1
Fatigue	1	2	1	<1
Diarrhea	1	1	<1	1
Rash	1	<1	0	0
Somnolence	1	<1	0	0
Flushing	1	2	<1	<1
Hyperuricemia	<1	2	2	1
Urinary frequency	<1	1	<1	1
Dry mouth	<1	1	1	0
SGPT increased	<1	1	1	1

* The order of AEs is based on their overall frequency (highest to lowest) in the moexipril group.

Table 6.2: Adverse events (in %) occurring in placebo-controlled moexipril studies*.

Adverse events	Moexipril n = 1355	Moexipril/ HCTZ n = 604	HCTZ n = 327	Placebo n = 417
Headache	11	7	7	12
Upper respiratory infection	8	4	4	7
Cough	7	5	1	3
Vertigo	5	3	2	2
Pain	4	2	3	4
Diarrhoea	4	3	2	1
Flu syndrome	4	3	1	1
Rhinitis	4	1	1	4
Fatigue	3	4	2	1
Sinusitis	2	1	1	2
Pharyngitis	2	2	1	1
Back pain	2	1	1	3
Dyspepsia	2	1	0	1
Nausea	2	1	1	1
Peripheral oedema	2	1	0	2
Rash	2	1	1	1
Hypokalaemia	<1	2	1	0
Hyperuricaemia	<1	3	3	1

* Judged not necessarily to be related to the drug.

dosage within the range of 3.75 mg to 60 mg. Serious adverse events, which did not always result in the discontinuation of a study, were seen in 2.3% of all the patients treated with moexipril.

Discontinuation of therapy because of adverse experiences was required in 4.3% of patients treated with moexipril and in 5.8% of patients treated with placebo. The most common reasons for discontinuation in patients treated with moexipril were cough (0.1%) and dizziness (0.2%).

All adverse experiences considered at least possibly related to treatment that ocurred at any dose in placebo-controlled trials in more than 1% of patients treated with moexipril alone and that were at least as frequent in the moexipril group as on placebo are shown in Table 6.2. Other adverse events occuring in more than 1% of patients on moexipril, but were at least as frequent on placebo include headache, upper respiratory infection, rhinitis, dyspepsia, nausea, peripheral edema, sinusitis, chest pain, and hyperuricemia. Cough was present in 7% of moexipril patients and 3% of patients given placebo. First dose hypotension, defined as a decrease in two minute SSBP of ≥ 30 mmHg, was observed in 8.1 and in 11.8% of patients receiving 7.5 and 15 mg moexipril, respectively. Only one of these patients was symptomatic.

Other adverse effects that have been reported with other ACE-inhibitors have also been observed with moexipril: angioedema or facial edema ($< 0.5\%$), hyp-

Table 6.3: Adverse events (in %) during long-term therapy with either moexipril or moexipril/HCTZ*.

	Moexipril n = 861	Moexipril/HCTZ n = 306
Adverse events	Figures in %	
Headache	12	8
Cough	10	12
Upper respiratory infections	12	17
Pain	9	12
Rhinitis	7	6
Dizziness	6	7
Back pain	5	6
Fatigue	5	3
Diarrhea	4	5
Pharyngitis	4	8
Sinusitis	4	5
Flu syndrome	3	8
Infection	2	5

* Judged not necessarily to be related to the drug.

erkalemia (0.8%), and minor increases in blood urea nitrogen (BUN) or creatinine (0.4%). Increases of BUN or creatinine are more likely to occur in patients receiving concomitant diuretics than in those on moexipril alone, and in patients with compromised renal function.

Although severe neutropenia did not occur in patients treated with moexipril, as with other ACE-inhibitors, monitoring of white blood cell counts should be considered for patients who have collagen-vascular disease, especially if the disease is associated with impaired renal function. Available data from clinical trials of moexipril are insufficient to show that moexipril does not cause agranulocytosis at rates similar to captopril (3, 30). Table 6.3 summarizes adverse experiences reported in uncontrolled long-term trials with a frequency of more than 3%.

Dosage and administration

Moexipril has shown to be an effective antihypertensive agent at doses from 7.5 mg to 60 mg administered once daily (13; data on file, Schwarz Pharma). All dosages have been well-tolerated and there was no relationship between dose and the incidence of adverse experiences. – Patients should begin treatment with moexipril 7.5 mg once daily. The usual dose is 7.5 mg to 15 mg once daily. Some patients will benefit from a further increase in dose to 30 mg once daily. However, doses above 30 mg do not produce any clinically relevant increase in efficacy. Few patients may respond better to moexipril if the total daily dose is given as two divided doses. In patients not sufficiently responding to moexipril monotherapy, a thiazide diuretic may be added. As add-on therapy to a diuretic in patients whose blood pressure is not sufficiently controlled by monotherapy the dosage of moexipril should be started with 7.5 mg.

In elderly patients and in other patients where an increased sensitivity to treatment with a drug that lowers peripheral resistance is to be expected, 7.5 mg moexipril once daily should be the initial dose. Patients with renal failure and liver failure should be started on 3.75 mg once daily. To avoid unnecessarily high dosages, it is recommended not to increase moexipril dosage too early. As with other ACE-inhibitors, maximal effects of a moexipril dose regimen are sometimes not seen before three to four weeks of treatment (23, 31). Moexipril is contraindicated in patients with a history of angioneurotic oedema, and should not be administered to children, pregnant or breastfeeding women. As with other ACE-inhibitors, moexipril should not be administered concomitantly with potassium salts or potassium-sparing diuretics, because of the increased risk of hyperkalemia, or with non-steroidal anti-inflammatory agents, which may attenuate the antihypertensive effect of ACE-inhibitors (3, 4, 23).

Summary

Moexipril is a new non-sulfhydryl angiotensin converting enzyme inhibitor, which has been developed for the once-daily treatment of essential hypertension. Moexipril in dosages of 7.5–30 mg alone or in combination with HCTZ, verapamil or nifedipine has shown to be an effective antihypertensive agent in patients with mild to moderate and moderate to severe hypertension. As compared to verapamil and HCTZ once-daily or captopril twice-daily, moexipril was as efficacious in mild to moderate hypertension. No development of tolerance was observed after long-term treatment of up to two years. No significant difference in the antihypertensive efficacy of moexipril could be detected between male and female patients with hypertension. The adverse reactions are as expected for an ACE-inhibitor, i. e. cough, headache and dizziness without evidence of a clear relationship between dose and incidence. No adverse event attributed to moexipril occurred that had not been reported previously for other ACE-inhibitiors. The usual dose is 7.5 mg to 15 mg moexipril once-daily.

Moexipril represents a valuable additon to the presently available ACE-inhibitors. Its use is facilitated by its potency and prolonged duration of action permitting a once-daily dosing schedule. Its efficacy in the treatment of primary hypertension is established.

In addition to the development program, which was performed in approximately 40% female and 60% male hypertensive patients, a number of studies was started in 1992 to establish the safety and efficacy of moexipril in postmenopausal women with hypertension, a subpopulation, which had been neglected in cardiovascular trials until recently. Some of the clinical and basic research data from this program, which was named the MADAM-program (**M**oexipril **A**s **A**ntihypertensive **D**rug **A**fter **M**enopause), have already been published (32–35) or are published in these proceedings.

References

1. The CONSENSUS Study Trial Group. Effects of enalapril on mortality in severe congestive heart failure. Results of the North Scandinavian enalapril survival study (CONSENSUS). N Engl J Med 1987; 316: 1429–1435.
2. The SOLVD Investigators. Effect of enalapril on survival in patients with reduced ventricular ejection fraction and congestive heart failure. N Engl J Med 1991; 325: 293–302.
3. Girard M. The safety of angiotensin-converting enzyme (ACE) inhibitiors in moderate hypertension. Adverse Drug React Toxicol Rev 1991; 10: 169–185.
4. Parish RC, Miller LJ. Adverse effects of angiotensin converting enzyme (ACE) inhibitors. An update. Drug Safety 1992; 7: 14–31.
5. Bafour JA, Goa KL. Benazepril: A review of its pharmacodynamic and pharmacokinetic properties, and therapeutic efficacy in hypertension and congestive heart failure. Drugs 1991; 42: 511–539.

6. Singhvi SM, Duchin KL, Morrision RA Willard DA, Everett DW, Frantz M. Disposition of fosinopril sodium in healthy subjects. Br J Clin Pharmacol 1988; 25: 9–15.
7. Lancaster SG, Todd PA: Lisinopril a preliminary review of its pharmacodynamic and pharmacokinetic properties and therapeutic use in hypertension and congestive heart failure. Drugs 1988; 35: 646–669.
8. Stimpel M, Cawello W. Pharmacokinetics and ACE-inhibition of the new ACE-inhibitor moexipril: Is Coadministration with food of clinical relevance? Hypertension 1995; 26: 1384.
9. Hui KK, Duchin KL, Kripalani KJ, Chan D, Kramer PK, Yanagawa N. Pharmacokinetics of fosinopril in patients with various degrees of renal function. Clin Pharmacol Ther 1991; 49: 457–467.
10. Todd PA, Benfield P. Ramipril: a review of its pharmacological properties and therapeutic use in cardiovascular disorders. Drugs 1990; 39: 110–135.
11. Edling O, Bao G, Feelisch M, Unger T, Gohlke P. Moexipril, a new angiotensin converting enzyme (ACE) inhibitor: Pharmacological characterization and comparison with enalapril. J Pharmacol Exp Ther 1995; 275: 854–863.
12. Stimpel M, Bonn R, Koch B, Dickstein K. Pharmacology and clinical use of the new ACE-inhibitor moexipril. Cardiovasc Drug Rev 1995; 13: 211–229.
13. Drayer JI, Stimpel M, Fox AAL, Weber MA. The antihypertensive properties of the angiotensin converting inhibitor moexipril given alone or in combination with a low dose of a diuretic. Am J Therap 1995; 2: 525- 531.
14. Persson B, Stimpel M. Evaluation of the antihypertensive efficacy and tolerability of moexipril, a new ACE inhibitor, compared to hydrochlorothiazide in elderly patients. Europ J Clin Pharmacol 1996; 50: 259–264.
15. Mroczek WJ, Stimpel M. A double-blind evaluation of moexipril versus hydrochlorothiazide in hypertension. Adv Ther 1996; 13: 79–87.
16. Lucas CP, Darga LL, Fox AAL, Stimpel M. A study of the efficacy and safety of moexipril in mild to moderate hypertension. Am J Therap 1995; 2: 886–892.
17. White WB, Whelton A, Fox AAL, Stimpel M, Kaihlanen PM. Tri-center assessment of the efficacy and pharmacodynamics of the ACE inhibitor, moexipril, by ambulatory blood pressure monitoring. J Clin Pharmacol 1995; 35: 233–238.
18. Koch B, Stimpel M, O. Andersson. Low-dose combinations of moexipril and hydrochlorothiazide in the treatment of hypertension. Pharmacol Res 1995; 31 (suppl.): 328.
19. Dickstein K, Aarsland T, Ferrari P, Todd M, Stimpel M. Comparison of the efficacy of three dose levels of moexipril versus placebo as add-on therapy to hydrochlorothiazide in patients with moderate hypertension. J Cardiovasc Pharmacol 1994; 24: 247–255.
20. Persson B, Widgren BR, Fox AAL, Stimpel M. Antihypertensive effects of moexipril, a new ACE inhibitor, as add on therapy to nifedipine in patients with essential hypertension. J Cardiovasc Pharmacol 1995; 26: 73–78.
21. Stimpel M, Loh IK. Moexipril versus Captopril in patients with mild to moderate hypertension. Am J Hypertension 1995; 8: 183 A.
22. Abernethy DR, Fox AAL, Stimpel M. Moexipril in the treatment of mild to moderate essential hypertension: comparison with sustained release verapamil. J Clin Pharmacol 1995; 35: 795–799.
23. Stimpel M. Inhibitors of the renin-angiotensin system. In Stimpel M: Arterial hypertension. Walter de Gruyter, Berlin-New York, 1996: 241–251.
24. White WB, Koch B, Stimpel M. Usefulness of moexipril and hydrochlorothiazide in moderately severe essential hypertension. Am J Therap 1996; 3: In press.
25. Koch B, Stimpel M. Do hypertensive women respond differently to low dosages of moexipril and hydrochlorothiazide? Hypertension 1995; 26: 1383.
26. White WB, Fox AAL, Stimpel M. Long-term efficacy and safety of moexipril in the treatment of hypertension. J Hum Hypertension 1994; 8: 17–921.

27. White WB, Stimpel M. Long-term safety and efficacy of moexipril alone and in combination with hydrochlorothiazide in elderly patients with hypertension. J Hum Hypertension 1995; 9: 879–884.
28. Chrysant SG, Fox AAL, Stimpel M. Comparison of moexipril – a novel ACE-inhibitor – to verapamil-SR as add-on therapy to low dose hydrochlorothiazide in hypertensive patients. Am J Hypertension 1995; 8: 418–421.
29. Saunders E, Weir MR, Kong W, Hollifield J, Gray J et al: A comparison of the efficacy and safety of a alpha-blocker, a calcium channel blocker, and a converting enzyme inhibitor in hypertensive blacks. Arch Intern Med 1990; 150: 1707–1713.
30. Heel RC, Brogden RN, Speight TM, Avery GS: Captopril: a preliminary review of its pharmacological properties and therapeutic efficacy. Drugs 1980; 20: 409–452.
31. Brunner HR, Waeber B, Nussberger J: Angiotensin-converting enzyme inhibitors in arterial hypertension. In Messerli FH (ed): Cardiovascular Drug Therapy, 2nd edition. WB Saunders, Philadelphia, 1996: 690–711.
32. Stimpel M, Jee WSS, Ma Y, Yamamoto N, Chen Y. Impact of antihypertensive therapy on postmenopausal osteoporosis: effects of the angiotensin converting enzyme inhibitor moexipril, 17-β-estradiol and their combination on the ovariectomy-induced cancellous bone loss in young rats. J Hypertens 1995; 13: 1852–1856.
33. Hatton R, Stimpel M, Chambers TJ. Angiotensin II is generated from angiotensin I by bone cells and stimulates osteoclastic bone resorption in vitro. J Endocrinol; in press.
34. Stimpel M, Koch B. Antihypertensive treatment in postmenopausal women with hypertension and obesity: moexipril versus atenolol. Am J Hypertens 1996; 9: 179A.
35. Grohe C, Kahlert S, Löbbert K, van Eickels M, Stimpel M, Vetter H, Neyses L. Inhibition of estrogen-stimulated cardiac fibroblast growth by moexiprilat. Europ J Pharmacol; in press.

7 The treatment of hypertension in postmenopausal women: experience with moexipril

Michael A. Weber

Emerging issues in hypertension

The treatment of hypertension appears to provide clinical benefits in virtually all populations in whom it has been offered. Although treatment historically was directed mainly at patients with more severe forms of hypertension, it has become evident that even patients with modest increases in blood pressure can benefit from therapy. Moreover, evidence that antihypertensive treatment significantly reduces major clinical events in the elderly has further expanded the size of the hypertensive population eligible for treatment (1–3).

Recommendations by such groups of experts as the Joint National Committee on the Detection, Evaluation, and Treatment of High Blood Pressure in their recent fifth report (JNC V) reflect this more aggressive approach to diagnosis and treatment (4). Indeed, the JNC recommends that individuals aged 18 or older be classified as hypertensive if their systolic blood pressures are 140 mmHg or higher or if their diastolic blood pressures are 90 mmHg or higher. Not all patients with a diagnosis of mild hypertension will necessarily require drug therapy, but it is clear that a substantial proportion of the population, especially the elderly, will now require management of their hypertension. Quite obviously, postmenopausal women will constitute a major part of this hypertensive group.

If the goal of treating hypertension is to reduce blood pressure to an acceptable level, notably 140/90 mmHg or below, it must be acknowledged that our performance in the community as a whole – especially in the United States – has been disappointing. The findings of the National Health and Nutrition Examination Survey (NHANES 3), as discussed in the JNC V Report (4), showed that barely one-quarter of hypertensive patients had met this goal. Explanations for this apparently poor result have included inadequate diagnosis, loss of patients to follow-up, and inadequate patient compliance with treatment. But, in addition, much of the problem can be attributed to a failure by physicians to fully respond to the challenge of treating hypertension, especially in older patients. Again, postmenopausal women appear to be a critical group with unmet needs.

Postmenopausal women and hypertension

Because so much of this book deals with aspects of cardiovascular disease in postmenopausal women, it is not necessary here to justify the importance of the diagnosis and treatment of hypertension in these individuals. It should be stressed, however, that with the growing emphasis on the importance of systolic hypertension as a separate cardiovascular risk factor, more focus continues to be placed on managing hypertension in the elderly. In turn, it is important to recognize that the elderly are the most rapidly growing segment of our population, and that post-menopausal women constitute more than 50% of this group.

A pivotal finding in recent studies of older hypertensive patients, in particular the Systolic Hypertension in the Elderly Program (SHEP), is that women were shown to benefit just as strongly as men in terms of reduced cardiovascular events during antihypertensive treatment (1). This was an important discovery, for previously it had been conjectured that women might be less vulnerable than men to hypertensive risk factors, and thereby less likely to benefit from treatment. It would be wrong, though, to assume that the treatment of middle aged or older women should necessarily follow the same rules as those for men; for example, the question of ongoing hormone replacement therapy in postmenopausal clearly raises questions that must be addressed in deciding on appropriate strategies.

Therapeutic approaches: the emergence of ACE inhibitors

Before considering the major questions involved in providing optimal care for hypertensive postmenopausal women, it is important to evaluate contemporary approaches to therapy. Although there are several classes of effective antihypertensive drugs available, the agents most commonly now in use are the diuretics; the beta blockers; the calcium channel blockers; the angiotensin converting enzyme (ACE) inhibitors; and the selective alpha blockers. There are pros and cons regarding the utility of each of these drug types, and realistically they all play a part in allowing physicians to tailor an optimal treatment regimen for each individual patient.

The ACE inhibitors have continued to grow in use for the treatment of hypertension. Much of this change has be driven by arguments that these drugs may have cardiovascular benefits beyond their blood pressure-lowering properties (5). One compelling argument comes from observations in clinical trials in congestive heart failure (6), post-myocardial infarction (7), and such other conditions as diabetic renal disease in which it as been shown that the ACE inhibitors can reduce the incidence of new cardiovascular events (8). Although clinical trials of these agents in hypertensive patients are not yet completed, it already seems reasonable to assume that the ACE inhibitors will be more effective in reducing coronary events than the more traditional agents. In considering the treatment of postmenopausal women, in whom major coronary events are a frequent occurrence, these drugs would appear to be of particular relevance.

This article will briefly review (see below) experiences with a newly-available ACE inhibitor, moexipril, in the treatment of hypertension in postmenopausal women. Data will be examined from four separate studies that have employed this agent within this selected population. Previous experience with moexipril has demonstrated its antihypertensive efficacy (9–11). Figure 7.1 shows its ef-

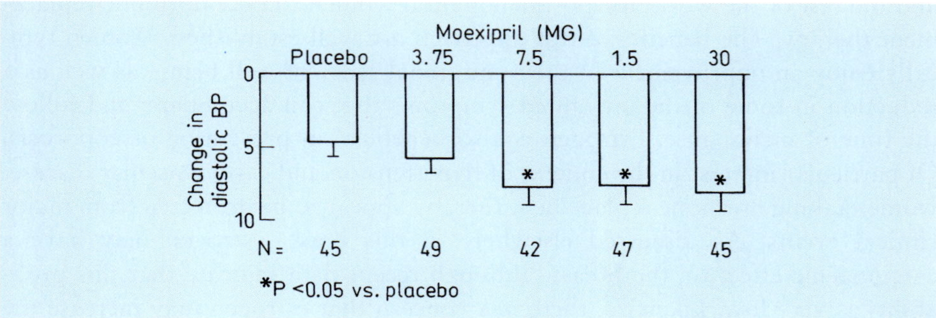

Figure 7.1: Effects of moexipril on diastolic blood pressure in patients with mild to moderate hypertension.

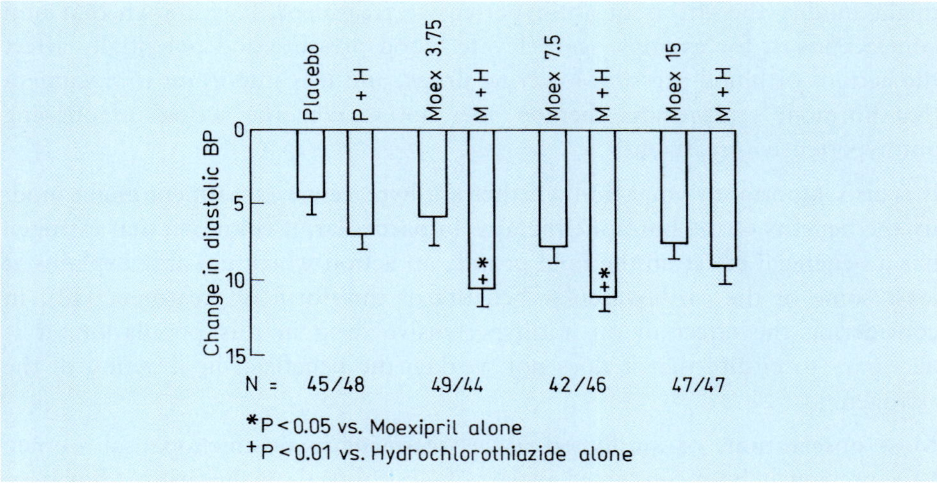

Figure 7.2: Effects of placebo (P), moexipril (M), and hydrochlorothiazide (H) on diastolic blood pressure in patients with mild to moderate hypertension.

fects on blood pressure in a group of men and women with mild-to-moderate hypertension (9). It is clear that once-daily doses of 7.5 mg or higher significantly reduce blood pressure at the end of the 24 hours dosing interval. It is also noteworthy that moexipril, as with other ACE inhibitors, works very effectively when combined with low doses of a diuretic. Figure 7.2 shows that a combination of low-dose moexipril with low-dose hydrochlorothiazide produces powerful antihypertensive effects.

Key questions

It is now commonplace in the United States and throughout much of Europe and the rest of the world for postmenopausal women to take hormone replacement therapy. The benefits of this approach are well established. Women typically enjoy an improvement in their emotional sense of well being, as well as a reduction in some of the unwanted symptoms that can accompany and follow the time of menopause. Estrogen is also beneficial in preventing osteoporosis. Of particular interest in the context of hypertension and cardiovascular disease, women taking hormone replacement therapy appear to be protected from major clinical events. As discussed elsewhere in this book, estrogen may have a carcinogenic effect on the breast, although recent data indicate that this probability is very low. Likewise, there is a concern that estrogen may increase the risk of uterine cancer, but concomitant administration of progesterone appears to prevent this adverse effect.

It becomes relevant, therefore, to ask whether hormone replacement therapy might modify the effects of antihypertensive treatment. It is known that oral contraceptives, for example, can elevate blood pressure and potentially affect the actions of blood pressure-lowering drugs, and it is important to document that hormone replacement therapy does not weaken the actions of ongoing antihypertensive treatment.

It is also important to question whether antihypertensive treatment might modify the benefits of the hormone therapy. In particular, it is known that estrogen has a beneficial effect on the lipid profile, an action which possibly explains at least some of the cardiovascular benefits of this form of treatment (12). In considering the effect of an antihypertensive drug in this population, it is necessary to ensure that it does not weaken the beneficial lipid action of the estrogen.

Most observations of antihypertensive treatment in postmenopausal women have previously been conducted as part of clinical trials evaluating cardiovascular endpoints in middle aged to elderly populations. As noted earlier, the postmenopausal women participating in these trials appeared to benefit to the same extent as men. Because these trials originated several years ago, for the most part before the more modern drugs now in use became available, much of this experience has been with diuretics and beta blockers. As yet, definitive outcome studies with ACE inhibitors have not been undertaken, and even the efficacy of this drug class has not been thoroughly studied in this particular population. For this reason, it becomes appropriate to ask whether ACE inhibitors are efficacious and safe in postmenopausal women.

It has been generally believed that the treatments of choice in middle aged or older hypertensive patients have been diuretics and calcium channel blockers. These two drugs classes are known to work well in the elderly, and possibly be more efficacious than in younger individuals. In contrast, ACE inhibitors have been considered the drugs of choice for younger individuals, perhaps because activity of the renin-angiotensin system is relatively greater in the young. In general, clinical experiences with ACE inhibitors have not really borne out this expectation, but careful examination of the usefulness of the ACE inhibitors in postmenopausal women clearly is warranted. It is certainly appropriate to compare the efficacy of these agents with other commonly used drugs, including representatives of the diuretic, beta blocker, and calcium channel blocker classes.

The following synopses of a series of recently completed studies will provide information that wholly or at least partly addresses this series of questions. It must be stressed that these results have not yet been published elsewhere, and that this report is preliminary in nature and does not present all the data that might subsequently become available.

Study 1: comparison of moexipril with placebo

This was a double-blind, randomized clinical trial carried out in multiple centers in the United States. The patients were postmenopausal women already taking hormone replacement therapy, which they continued throughout the study. The patients either had not previously been treated for hypertension or were free of treatment for at least four weeks prior to active treatment. Their baseline diastolic blood pressures were between 95 mmHg and 109 mmHg.

The treatment period lasted for twelve weeks. Patients were randomized to receive either moexipril (N = 43) or placebo (N = 36). The dose of moexipril in this study was 15 mg once daily.

The principal blood pressure results are shown in Table 7.1. Moexipril produced significant reductions in diastolic and systolic blood pressures, and the diastolic effect was significantly greater than that observed with the placebo.

Table 7.1: Treatment for 12 weeks in postmenopausal hypertensive women taking hormone replacement therapy.

	Diastolic BP		Systolic BP	
	Moexipril N = 43	Placebo N = 36	Moexipril N = 43	Placebo N = 36
Baseline	99.5	100.0	154.6	158.5
Decrease	9.9*	4.3*	12.2*	1.6

Dose: Moexipril 15 mg daily. *$P < 0.001$; also, decrease in diastolic BP greater with moexipril ($P = 0.016$) than placebo. Values are mean of seated BP.

One of the major goals of this study was to observe metabolic measurements during antihypertensive treatment in patients receiving hormone replacement therapy. No changes in key measurements were observed during moexipril treatment. Average fasting plasma glucose was 94 mg/dL at baseline, and 94.5 mg/dL at the end of the study in the moexipril group. Likewise HDL-cholesterol was unchanged with moexipril, being 64 mg/dL both at the beginning and end of the treatment period. The total cholesterol/HDL ratio was 3.7 both at the beginning and end of moexipril treatment. It was also noted that there was a small reduction in fibrinogen from 322 mg/dL to 288 mg/dL, and a small increase in plasminogen activator inhibitor from 14.8 mg/dL to 15.7 mg/dL with moexipril therapy. Neither of these changes in clotting measurements reached significance. Similarly, there were no changes in any of these measurements in the placebo group.

Symptomatic adverse events reported during the study were 33/47 in the moexipril group, and 28/48 in the placebo group. Clearly, there was no significant difference between the groups. Thus, this study demonstrated that moexipril produced significant blood pressure-lowering effects in postmenopausal women on hormone replacement therapy, without evidence for meaningful adverse effects. The moexipril treatment also did not alter the principal metabolic measurements in these women receiving hormone replacement therapy.

Study 2: comparison of moexipril with atenolol

This was a double-blind, randomized clinical trial conducted at multiple centers in the United States. The patients were postmenopausal women who were recruited into the study regardless of whether or not they were taking hormone replacement therapy. The patients had either never been treated for hypertension or were free of antihypertensive treatment for at least fours weeks prior to the start of active study therapy. At baseline, the patients had seated diastolic blood pressures between 95 mmHg and 109 mmHg. Because of the interest in pursuing metabolic issues, it was decided to conduct this study in women who were considered to be obese on the basis of weighing more than their ideal body weights at least 30%.

This was a 12 week study. Patients were randomized to receive either moexipril (N = 58) or the beta blocker atenolol (N = 58). The starting dose of moexipril was 7.5 mg once daily. If, after 4 weeks of treatment, diastolic blood pressure remained at 90 mmHg or above, the dose was doubled to 15 mg once daily for the rest of the study. The starting dose of atenolol was 25 mg once daily, and this was titrated to 50 mg once daily if the response was not adequate at 4 weeks.

The principal blood pressure findings from this study are shown in Table 7.2. Both moexipril and atenolol significantly decreased diastolic and systolic blood pressures. Although the moexipril tended to be slightly more efficacious than the atenolol, this difference was not significant.

Table 7.2: Treatment in obese postmenopausal women.

	Diastolic BP		Systolic BP	
	Moexipril N = 58	Atenolol N = 58	Moexipril N = 58	Atenolol N = 58
Baseline	101.5	100.7	159.5	154.5
Decrease	10.4*	8.4*	14.7*	8.7*

Doses: Moexipril 7.5 or 15 mg, Atenolol 25 or 50 mg. *$P < 0.001$. Values are mean of seated BP. Patients were 30 to 80% above ideal body weight.

There were no differences between the two drugs in reported symptomatic adverse events. It was noted, however, that following randomization the patients assigned to moexipril were heavier (94.5 kg) than those assigned to atenolol (89.5 kg). In general neither drug produced meaningful changes in metabolic measurements. The one value of note, however, was the glycosylated hemoglobin (HbA_{1C}) which increased significantly ($P < 0.02$) in the atenolol group, but did not change in the moexipril group.

This experience demonstrated that the ACE inhibitor moexipril was efficacious in postmenopausal women despite their increased body weight. Because of the high prevalence of obesity in our society, this finding appears to be of practical importance.

Study 3: comparison of moexipril with hydrochlorothiazide

This was a double-blind, randomized clinical trial conducted in several centers within the United States. The patients were postmenopausal women who were recruited into the study regardless of whether or not they were on hormone replacement therapy. The patients either had never been treated for hypertension or were free of antihypertensive therapy for at least 4 weeks prior to receiving active study treatment. Their baseline diastolic blood pressures were between 95 mmHg and 109 mmHg.

Patients were randomized to receive either moexipril (N = 43) or hydrochlorothiazide (N = 41). Throughout this 12 week study the dose of moexipril was 15 mg once daily, and the dose of hydrochlorothiazide was 25 mg once daily.

The principal effects of these drugs on blood pressure are shown in Table 7.3. Each drug significantly reduced both the diastolic and systolic blood pressures. Although the effects of these drugs on lipid measurements were not significantly different from each other, there were two other metabolic measurements of interest. Uric acid increased more (P = 0.01) with hydrochlorothiazide (from 4.9 mg/dL to 5.7 mg/dL) than with moexipril (4.8 mg/dL to 4.9 mg/dL). Similarly, plasma glucose concentrations increased with hydrochlorothiazide (+11.0 mg/dL, P = 0.011), but did not change with moexipril (−2.4 mg/dL). Although both drugs were well tolerated, there was a tendency for symptomatic adverse events to be reported more commonly with hydrochlorothiazide (53.1%) than with moexipril (39.6%).

Table 7.3: Treatment for 12 weeks in postmenopausal women.

	Diastolic BP		Systolic BP	
	Moexipril N = 43	HCTZ N = 41	Moexipril N = 43	HCTZ N = 41
Baseline	100.5	100.5	159.0	158.8
Decrease	10.0*	11.8*	8.0*	15.5*

Doses: Moexipril 15 mg daily, HCTZ 25 mg daily. *P < 0.001. Values are mean of seated BP.

These findings again confirm that moexipril as monotherapy significantly reduces blood pressure in postmenopausal women. It also points out that the diuretic hydrochlorothiazide, even in a relatively low 25 mg dose, significantly increases both uric acid and glucose plasma concentrations. These issues may be of importance in reviewing the overall cardiovascular risk profile in postmenopausal patients.

Study 4: comparison of moexipril with nitrendipine

This was a double-blind, randomized clinical trial conducted at several centers within Europe. The patients were postmenopausal women who were recruited regardless of whether or not they were taking hormone replacement therapy. The patients either had never been treated for hypertension or had been free of antihypertensive therapy for at least 4 weeks prior to the start of active study treatment. Their baseline diastolic blood pressures were in the range 95 mmHg to 109 mmHg.

Patients were randomized to receive either moexipril (N = 45) or nitrendipine (N = 47). The dose of moexipril was 15 mg once daily throughout the study, and the dose of nitrendipine was 20 mg daily. Unlike the other studies, which were 12 weeks in duration, this study provided active treatment for 8 weeks.

The principal blood pressure effects of the two drugs are shown in Table 7.4. Moexipril and nitrendipine each significantly reduced both diastolic and systolic blood pressures. There was a trend for moexipril to be slightly more efficacious than nitrendipine, but this difference was not significant.

Table 7.4: Treatment for 8 weeks in postmenopausal hypertensive women.

	Diastolic BP		Systolic BP	
	Moexipril N = 45	Nitrendipine N = 47	Moexipril N = 45	Nitrendipine N = 47
Baseline	103.0	102.3	161.3	162.2
Decrease	15.2*	13.6*	21.2*	18.2*

Doses: Moexipril 15 mg daily, nitrendipine 20 mg daily. *P < 0.001. Values are mean of seated Bp.

There were no significant differences between the two drugs in their metabolic effects. There were differences, however, in symptomatic complaints. Nitrendipine was more likely than moexipril to produce headache (P = 0.014) and ankle edema (P = 0.012). Predictably, moexipril was somewhat more likely than nitrendipine to produce cough (P = 0.053). For overall adverse events, the incidence was significantly greater with nitrendipine than with moexipril (P = 0.0027).

This study shows the comparability of the ACE inhibitor with the calcium channel blocker, even in a group of postmenopausal women who might be regarded as strong candidates for calcium channel blocker therapy. The adverse events were typical for the two drug classes; calcium channel blockers, especially dihydropyridines, are known to produce ankle edema and headache, whereas ACE inhibitors have a tendency to cause cough.

Conclusions

This short series of studies represents the first systematic attempt to study a new drug in an important hypertensive population, postmenopausal women. As is discussed in depth throughout this book, we have only recently come to recognize that this important population has a cardiovascular risk profile and prognosis that has not been previously well studied or understood. For this reason, it cannot simply be assumed that drugs which work well in a younger group of patients, or in a population drawn mainly from male hypertensives, will be appropriate in postmenopausal women.

Taken together, these experiences with moexipril have demonstrated that this ACE inhibitor works effectively as an antihypertensive agent regardless of whether or not postmenopausal patients are taking hormone therapy. Indeed, in the placebo-controlled study, in which all the patients were receiving hormone replacement therapy, the effects of the drug were similar to those observed previously in other study populations (9–11). Thus, it seems improbable that hormone replacement therapy creates any resistance to the blood pressure effects of this ACE inhibitor.

It was also clear from these studies that moexipril demonstrated efficacy that is comparable to other widely used drug classes. Although ACE inhibitors previously had been considered to be most efficacious in younger patients, these new studies indicate that moexipril performs similarly to the diuretic, hydrochlorothiazide, and the calcium channel blocker, nitrendipine, in a more mature patient group. Moexipril also showed that it was at least as effective as the beta blocker atenolol. These findings indicate that moexipril, from an efficacy point of view, represents a very strong alternative to other drug classes in treating postmenopausal hypertensive women.

One of the key attributes of ACE inhibitors that has led to their wide use is that they produce remarkably few unwanted side effects. This was clearly the finding in this recent group of studies. Indeed, there was a suggestion that the incidence of patient complaints was lower with moexipril than with either the calcium channel blocker or the diuretic. Of course, side effects are a problem for individual patients, and it is usually not possible to predict which patient will be tolerant of a particular drug class. Complaints such as ankle edema and headache tend to occur more commonly with calcium channel blockers than with other drug classes, whereas ACE inhibitors are more prone to cause cough. Diuretics and beta blockers also are not free of adverse effects. Overall, these findings indicate that moexipril is emerging as a well tolerated drug for this particular patient group.

These studies, of themselves, were not sufficiently powerful or rigorously conducted to fully evaluate metabolic measurements. Some interesting trends, though, did emerge. The diuretic, even in a relatively low dose, produced the expected increases in plasma concentrations of uric acid and glucose. The beta blocker tended to increase glycosolated hemoglobin, perhaps indicating an unwanted effect on glucose tolerance. Moexipril, as with other ACE inhibitors reported previously, appears to have no adverse effects on metabolic measurements. There has been some interest in the possibility that ACE inhibitors could influence clotting mechanisms, and we noted that moexipril slightly decreased fibrinogen and slightly increased plasminogen activator inhibitor. Neither of these changes was significant, and thus should not be over-interpreted. But it may be of interest to pursue these issues in more detail in the future.

What was of importance, in the metabolic context, was that moexipril did not adversely affect any of the glucose or lipid values in post-menopausal women already established on hormone replacement therapy. One of the apparent benefits of estrogen is that it favorably alters lipids (12), and it is reassuring to note that moexipril does not in any way dilute this positive attribute of the hormone replacement therapy.

In summary, moexipril now appears to be emerging as a desirable treatment for hypertension in postmenopausal women. It displays antihypertensive efficacy that compares favorably with other widely used antihypertensive drugs. It is well tolerated from a symptomatic point of view, and it potentially has some advantages, when compared with alternative drug classes, in avoiding unwanted metabolic effects. Hopefully, the brief studies reported herein will lead to further examination of this new approach to therapy in postmenopausal women.

References

1. Prevention of stroke by antihypertensive drug treatment in older persons with isolated "systolic hypertension: Funal results of the Systolic Hypertension in the Elderly Program "(SHEP). JAMA 1991; 265: 3255–3264.
2. Dahlof B, Lundholm L, Hansson L. et al: Morbidity and martality in the Swedish Trial in Old Patients with Hypertension (STOP-Hypertension). Lancet 1991; 338: 1281–1285.
3. MRC Working Party: Medical Research Council trial of treatment of hypertension in older adults: principal results: BMJ 1992; 304: 405–412.
4. Joint National Committee on Detection, Evaluation and Treatment of High Blood Pressure: Fifth Report (JNC V). Arch Intern Med 1993; 153: 154–183.
5. Weber MA, Laragh JH: Hypertension: steps forward and steps backward. Arch Intern Med 1993; 153: 149–152.
6. Cohn JN: The prevention of heart failure: A new agenda. N Engl J Med 1992; 327: 725–727.
7. Pfeffer, MA, Braunwald E, Moye LA, et al: Effect of captopril on mortality and morbidity in patients with left ventricular dysfunction after myocardial infarction. Results of the Survival and Ventricular Enlargement Trial. N Engl J Med 1992; 327: 669–677.
8. Lewis EJ, Hunsicker LG, Bain RP, Rohde RD, et al: The effect of angiotensin-converting-enzyme inhibition on diabetic nephropathy. N Engl J Med 1993; 329: 1456–1462.

9. Drayer JIM, Stimpel M, Fox A, Weber MA: The antihypertensive properties of the angiotensin converting enzyme inhibitor moexipril given alone or in combination with a low dose of a diuretic. Am J Therapeutics 1995; 2: 525–531.
10. White WB, Stimpel M: Long-term safety and efficacy of moexipril alone and in combination with hydrochlorothiazide in elderly patients with hypertension. J Hum Hypertens 1995; 9: 879–884.
11. White WB, Fox AL, Stimpel M: Long-term efficacy and safety of moexipril in the treatment of hypertension. J Hum Hypertens 1994; 8: 917–921.
12. Lobo RA: Effects of hormonal replacement in lipids and lipoproteins in postmenopausal women. J Clin Endocrinol Metab 1991; 73: 925.

8 Role of the renin-angiotensin system in the regulation of bone resorption

Timothy J. Chambers, Michael Stimpel,
Ruth Hatton

Throughout life, bone undergoes continuous resorption by osteoclasts and reformation by osteoblasts. These activities are normally integrated to the requirements of skeletal morphogenesis and restructuring, and to those of calcium homeostasis. Failure of integration of these activities to the role of bone as a structural support is seen in the loss of bone that leads to osteoporosis; the scale of the contribution of this dysregulation to disease is emphasised by the observation that 40% of all women over the age of 65 have suffered fractures of radius, vertebra or femur (1). Of the 30% who sustain a fractured femur by age 90, 27% die within the first year as a direct result of the fracture; the remainder are often rendered less mobile and more dependent (1).

The disease is much more common in females, in whom it is due to bone loss which starts at the menopause. Bone mass decreases by 2–5 per cent per annum after the menopause, so that by age 65, women have lost a considerable proportion of their bone.

The bone loss is due to estrogen deficiency. Similar bone loss is seen after ovariectomy in amenorrheic women and in other hypoestrogenic states (2–5). Estrogen normally exerts a suppressive effect on bone resorption and reduction in estrogen levels leads to increased bone resorption. During normal remodelling in bone, bone resorption and bone formation are in balance: an increase in bone resorption leads to an increase in bone formation. However, in estrogen deficiency, although bone formation does increase as a consequence of the increased resorption, the increase is insufficient to compensate fully for the increased resorption. Thus, estrogen causes bone loss through an increase in bone resorption, together with a relative deficiency in bone formation (6, 7).

The mechanism by which estrogen deficiency stimulates bone resorption is controversial. It has been suggested that there is increased osteoclast generation due to raised IL(interleukin)-1 or IL-6 production by bone marrow stromal cells (see 8, 9). Ultimately, however, bone resorption is likely to be controlled at the bone surface, at sites of resorption. We have found that estrogen does not inhibit osteoclastic bone resorption directly, but does so in co-cultures of osteoclasts with cells of the osteoblastic lineage (10). This observation is consistent with evidence that osteoblastic cells possess estrogen receptors (11, 12).

The above observations emphasise the close interdependency of the processes of bone resorption and bone formation, and of the osteoclasts and osteoblastic cells that mediate these processes. In fact, it is well recognised that cells of the osteoblastic series (including bone-forming osteoblasts, bone lining cells and osteocytes) exert a major influence over the resorptive activity of osteoclasts (see 13). This is evidenced, for example, in the lack of receptors for parathyroid hormone on osteoclasts, and their presence on osteoblasts. Thus, parathyroid hormone stimulates bone resorption not through an action on the resorptive cell itself, but through a primary interaction with osteoblastic cells, which then stimulate osteoclastic function. Presumably osteoclasts, essentially wandering cells, need instruction from resident bone cells, as to where bone resorption is appropriate.

Osteocytes and the cells lining bone surfaces seem well suited to determine localisation of osteoclastic activity. Osteocytes, embedded in bone, make extensive gap junctional communication with each other and with the bone surface via canaliculi. These cells seem likely not only to determine sites of bone resorption, appropriate for the morphogenesis and restructuring of bone, but also to determine where on bone surfaces bone formation is most appropriate. Consistent with this, osteocytes have recently been shown to be sensitive to mechanical stimulation (see 14). We and others have noted that the earliest response of bone to mechanical stimulation is seen in osteocytes, followed some days later by new bone formation (see 15, 16). In our experiments, c-fos expression was detected in osteocytes and bone lining cells of rat vertebrae within 30 mins after a brief episode of mechanical stimulation.

However, in the above experiments, we also noted strong c-fos expression in cortical blood vessels. Blood vessels can detect fluid flow, but the response was only seen in cortical vessels, suggesting that physiologic strains in bone amplify, or cortical endothelial cells are more sensitive to, fluid flow. This enhanced vascular response seems less likely to be of relevance to the physiology of vascular homeostasis, and may rather be a component of the mechanical responsiveness of bone: the mechanism by which bone adapts its structure to the prevailing mechanical environment. A similar model, whereby mechanical stimulation of bone induces fluid flow, from the medullary cavity to the cortex, past osteocytes, has been suggested to account for osteocytic responses to mechanical strain (17). Thus, not only osteoblastic cells, but vascular cells might participate in the regulation of bone formation and resorption.

In fact, the cell biology of bone resorption and formation has for long been intimately linked to that of the local vasculature (see 18). Thus, during endochrondral bone formation, vascularisation of the cartilage model is associated with direct contact between the advancing osteoclasts and adjacent capillary loops, such that resorption can be conceptualised as part of a process of vascular invasion. Subsequently, capillaries are observed immediately adjacent to osteoclasts at resorptive sites on bone surfaces, and follow osteoclasts into bone during Haversian remodelling of cortical bone. Intense vascularity is a common feature in states of excessive bone resorption. This proximity provides an opportunity for regulation of bone resorption by endothelial cells. Similarly, osteoblastic cells accompany the capillaries that invade cartilage rudiments and colonise the excavated surfaces. Throughout subsequent life, osteoblasts follow osteoclasts and vessels onto excavated surfaces to reform bone. While it is likely that bone cells themselves provide much of the information that regulates this remodelling activity, from another perspective osteoclasts can be seen as the tools of vascular invasion, and osteoblasts and the bone subsequently formed as a specialised form of perivascular tissue. From this perspective, our experimental observations might reasonably represent a participation by the vasculature in the environmental responsiveness of bone.

These observations are consistent with the profound effect of endothelial products such as prostaglandins (19, 20), nitric oxide (21, 22), endothelin (23) and platelet activating factor (24–26) on osteoclast function. However, while the actions of the former agents on bone resorption have been relatively well studied, the actions of another major regulator of vascular physiology, angiotensin II (Ang II), have not been investigated.

Ang II is produced as part of the renin angiotensin system (RAS) and is well recognized for its cardiovascular and fluid and electrolyte regulatory activities (27). The traditional RAS cascade involving renal renin, hepatic angiotensinogen and lung endothelial angiotensin converting enzyme (ACE) interacting to produce Ang II is largely responsible for these major functions. It is however becoming increasingly clear that Ang II has local actions not related to these systemic actions, including a role in angiogenesis (28, 29). In view of the role of osteoclasts in the vascularization of bone, and the proximity of endothelial cells and osteoclasts, and the ability of endothelial cells to generate Ang II, we therefore elected to assess the effects of Ang II on osteoclasts.

We found that Ang II strongly stimulates bone resorption by osteoclasts incubated on bone slices in the presence of osteoblastic cells. Osteoclasts incubated without added osteoblastic cells did not respond. This suggests that, in common with several other agents, stimulation of bone resorption by Ang II occurs not through a direct effect on osteoclasts, but is mediated by a primary hormornal interaction on cells of the osteoblastic lineage (see 13). Stimulation was significant at concentrations of Ang II of 10^{-7}M and above, and was similar in degree to that of the major calcium-regulating hormone, $1{,}25(OH)_2$ vitamin D_3. These results suggest that Ang II has the potential ability to play a physiologically-significant role in the regulation of osteoclastic bone resorption.

Generally, Ang I is converted to Ang II by ACE, present on the surface of endothelial cells (30, 31). In view of the proximity of osteoclasts to endothelial cells during bone resorption, the role of osteoclasts in vascularization, and the ability of endothelial cells to generate other agents that regulate osteoclast activity, it is possible that under physiologic circumstances, bone endothelial cells induce local bone destruction by production of Ang II, analagous to the role of Ang II in angiogenesis that has been proposed in the ovary (29). Ang II-induced osteolysis may be a component of the primary function of the systemic RAS, which is the regulation of the cardiovascular system and fluid and electrolyte physiology. Alternatively, Ang II might, as in the ovary, be a mediator of local tissue interactions, unrelated to the physiologic aims of the generalized RAS. In this case, a local source of Ang I would have to be postulated, as in the ovary, to enable interactions in bone to be independent of the regulation of the systemic RAS.

However, rather unexpectedly, we found that Ang I itself stimulated bone resorption in cocultures of osteoclasts with osteoblastic cells. This stimulation was inhibited by the ACE inhibitor moexiprilat, suggesting that conversion of Ang I to Ang II by ACE was responsible for the stimulation of bone resorption. Thus, while it remains possible that endothelial cells are able to regulate osteoclastic bone resorption through Ang II generation, the requirement of osteoblastic cells as an intermediary in this stimulation, coupled with the ability of osteoblast-osteoclast cultures to themselves generate Ang II, implies that the system might also be a mechanism for regulation of bone resorption intrinsic to bone cells themselves.

Although the RAS is well documented in the regulation of the cardiovascular system, it is becoming increasingly clear that the components of the system have a wider distribution than previously envisaged, and in some cases at least, have a physiologic function independent of systemic vascular control. Thus, messenger RNAs for both renin and angiotensinogen are expressed in the kidney and also in cells of the adrenal, brain, heart, and reproductive tissues (32–36); Ang II receptors have been found not only in vascular tissue and other systemic targets of the RAS, but also in pancreatic acinar and ductal cells (37, 38), ovarian follicular epithelial cells (39–42), the mesenchyme surrounding developing cartilage (43, 44), and in hepatocytes (45) and fibroblasts (46, 47); and ACE has been reported in not only endothelial cells but also in fibroblasts (48, 49), activated macrophages (50); ovarian follicular epithelium (40) and in sperm, where the enzyme is crucial to fertility (51).

Our results suggest that it is not necessary to invoke endothelial cell participation in regulation of bone resorption by the RAS. Nevertheless, there are striking parallels between the effects of endothelial and bone cell signals on bone physiology. Thus, both osteoblastic and endothelial cells have been reported to be able to induce osteoclast differentiation (52, 53). Nitric oxide is produced by endothelial (see 54) and osteoblastic cells (55), and causes vasodilatation (56), suppression of bone resorption (21, 22) and plays a role in the induction of bone formation (57). Similarly, prostaglandin is produced by both cells types, and is a vasodilator that has anti-resorptive properties (20), and is implicated in osteogenesis (see 58). Ang II appears to show a corresponding pattern, acting as vasoconstrictor and osteolytic agent. These parallel patterns of responsiveness might reflect mechanisms that developed to co-ordinate bone physiology with angiogenesis. Whatever the evolutionary origin of the actions of Ang I and II, our data identify Ang I and Ang II as potent regulators of osteoclastic bone resorption, and raise the possibility that bone contains a tissue RAS. To establish this, and to assess its role in physiology, it will be necessary to identify the sites, and regulation of expression, of the components of this system in bone.

A further implication of these results is that ACE inhibitors, including moexiprilat, might suppress bone resorption in vivo, an action that might be of value when such inhibitors are used in the treatment of hypertension in postmenopausal women. One study in rats (59), using a well-established model for the osteoporosis of estrogen deficiency, found that ACE inhibition by moexipril has no effect on the skeleton when given alone, and that it does not hamper the osteoprotective effects of 17β-estradiol. However, this study had a number of limitations. Only one dose was used; and effects might be different in hypertensive compared to normotensive states; it might be more difficult to detect an effect of ACE inhibition on the rapid and substantial bone loss of ovariectomized rats than on the more gradual bone loss in postmenopausal women. Thus, while the available evidence makes it unlikely that ACE-inhibitors would potentiate postmenopausal bone loss, their potential for osteoprotection remains unknown.

References

1. Royal College of Physicians. Fractured neck of femur: prevention and management. A report of the Royal College of Physicians. London: Royal College of Physicians, 1989.
2. Schlechter JA, Sherman R, Martin R. Bone density in amenorrheic women with and without hyperprolactinemia. J Clin Endocrinol Metab 1983; 56: 1120–1123.
3. Cann CE, Martin MC, Genant HK, Jaffe RB. Decreased spinal mineral content in amenorrheic women. J Am Med Assn 1984; 251: 626–629.
4. Koppelman MCS, Kurtz DW, Morrish KA, et al. Vertebral body bone mineral content in hyperprolactinemic women. J Clin Endocrinol Metab 1984; 59: 1050–1053.
5. Rigotti NA, Nussbaum SR, Herzog DB, Neer RM. Osteoporosis in women with anorexia nervosa. N Engl J Med 1984; 311: 1601–1606.
6. Christiansen C, Christiansen MS, Larsen N-E, Transbol I. Pathophysiological mechanism of estrogen effect on bone metabolism: dose-response relationship in early postmenopausal women. J Clin Endocrinol Metab 1982; 55: 1124–1130.
7. Steiniche T, Hasling C, Charles P, Eriksen EF, Mosekilde L, Melsen F. A randomised study on the effects of estrogen/gestagen or high dose oral calcium on trabecular bone remodeling in postmenopausal osteoporosis. Bone 1989; 10: 313–320.

8. Kimble RB, Vannice JL, Bloedow DC, et al. Interleukin-1 receptor antagonist decreases bone loss and bone resorption in ovariectomized rats. J Clin Invest 1994; 93: 1959–1967.
9. Jilka RL, Hangoc G, Girasole G, et al. Increased osteoclast development after estrogen loss: Mediation by interleukin-6. Science 1992; 257: 88–91.
10. Tobias JH, Chambers TJ. Effect of sex hormones on bone resorption by rat osteoclasts. Acta Endocrinol 1991; 124: 121–127.
11. Ernst M, Heath JK, Rodan GA. Estradiol effects on proliferation, messenger ribonucleic acid for collagen and insulin-like growth factor-I, and parathyroid hormone-stimulated adenylate cyclase activity in osteoblastic cells from calvariae and long bones. Endocrinology 1989; 125: 825–833.
12. Komm BS, Terpening CM, Benz DJ, et al. Estrogenic binding, receptor mRNA and biologic response in osteoblast-like osteosarcoma cells. Science 1988; 241: 81–84.
13. Chambers TJ. Regulation of osteoclast development and function. In: Rifkin BR, Gay CV, eds. Biology and Physiology of the Osteoclast. Boca Raton: CRC Press, 1992; 105–128.
14. Klein-Nulend J, van der Plas A, Semeins CM, et al. Sensitivity of osteocytes to biomechanical stress in vitro. FASEB J 1995; 9: 441–445.
15. Skerry TM, Bitensky L, Chayen J, Lanyon LE. Early strain-related changes in enzyme activity in osteocytes following bone loading in vivo. J Bone Min Res 1989; 4(5): 783–788.
16. Lean J, Jagger C, Chambers T, Chow J. Increased insulin-like growth factor I mRNA expression in rat osteocytes in response to mechanical stimulation. Am J Physiol 1995; 268: E318–E327.
17. Hillsley MV, Frangos JA. Review: Bone tissue engineering: The role of interstitial fluid flow. Biotech Bioeng 1994; 43: 573–581.
18. Streeten EA, Brandi ML. Biology of bone endothelial cells. Bone & Min 1990; 10: 85–94.
19. Klein DC, Raisz LG. Prostaglandins: stimulation of bone resorption in tissue culture. Endocrinology 1970; 86: 1436–1440.
20. Chambers TJ, McSheehy PMJ, Thomson BM, Fuller K. The effect of calcium-regulating hormones and prostaglandins on bone resorption by osteoclasts disaggregated from neonatal rabbit bones. Endocrinology 1985; 116: 234–239.
21. Brandi ML, Hukkanen M, Umeda T, et al. Bidirectional regulation of osteoclast function by nitric oxide synthase isoforms. Proc Natl Acad Sci USA 1995; 92: 2954–2958.
22. Kasten TP, Collin-Osdoby P, Patel N, et al. Potentiation of osteoclast bone-resorption activity by inhibition of nitric oxide synthase. Proc Natl Acad Sci USA 1994; 91: 3569–3573.
23. Zaidi M, Alam ASMT, Bax BE, et al. Role of the endothelial cell in osteoclast control: New perspectives. Bone 1993; 14: 97–102.
24. Wood DA, Hapak LK, Sims SM, Dixon SJ. Direct effects of PAF on isolated rat osteoclasts. J Biol Chem 1991; 266(23): 15369–15376.
25. Zheng ZG, Wood DA, Sims SM, Dixon SJ. PAF stimulates resorption by rabbit osteoclasts in vitro. Am J Physiol 1993; 264: E74–E81.
26. Wucherpfennig AL, Dewhirst FE, Stashenko P. PAF increases intracellular calcium in isolated osteoclasts but does not modify bone resorption. Bone 1993; 14: 13–18.
27. Peach MJ. Molecular actions of angiotensin. Biochem Pharmacol 1981; 30: 2745–2751.
28. Fernandez LA, Tarlatzis BC, Rzasa PJ, et al. Renin-like activity in ovarian follicular fluid. Fertil Steril 1985; 44: 219–223.
29. Andrade-Gordon P, Zreik T, Apa R, Naftolin F. Role of angiotensin II in the processes leading to ovulation. Biochem Pharmacol 1991; 42(4): 715–719.
30. Caldwell PRB, Seegal BC, Hsu KC, Das M, Soffer RL. Angiotensin-converting enzyme: vascular endothelial localization. Science 1976; 191: 1050–1051.
31. Takada Y, Hiwada K, Unno M, Kokubu T. Immunocytochemical localization of angiotensin converting enzyme at the ultrastructural level in the human lung and kidney. Biomed Res 1982; 3: 169–174.

32. Ganong WF. Origin of the angiotensin II secreted by cells. Proc Soc Exp Biol Med 1994; 205(3): 213–219.
33. Dzau VJ, Ellison KE, Brody T, Ingelfinger J, Pratt RE. A comparative study of the distribution of renin and angiotensinogen messenger ribonucleic acids in rat and mouse tissues. Endocrinology 1987; 120: 2334–2338.
34. Dzau VJ, Re RN. Evidence for the existence of renin in the heart. Circulation 1987; 75 (suppl II): II34-II36.
35. Samani NJ, Swales D, Brammer WJ. Expression of the renin gene in extra-renal tissues of the rat. Biochem J 1988; 253: 907–910.
36. Sealey JE, Laragh JH. The renin-angiotensin-aldosterone system for normal regulation of blood pressure and sodium and potassium homeostasis. In: Laragh JH, Brenner BM, eds. Hypertension: pathophysiology, diagnosis and management. New York: Raven Press, 1990; 1027–1317.
37. Chappell MC, Diz DI, Jacobsen DW. Pharmacological characterization of angiotensin II binding sites in the canine pancreas. Peptides 1992; 13: 313–318.
38. Chappell MC, Millsted A, Diz DI, Brosnihan KB, Ferrario CM. Evidence for an intrinsic angiotensin system in the canine pancreas. J Hypertens 1991; 9: 751–759.
39. Lightman A, Jones CL, McClusky NJ, Palumbo A, DeCherney AH, Naftolin F. Immunocytochemical localization of angiotensin II – Immunoreactivity and demonstration of angiotensin II binding in the rat ovary. Am J Obstet Gynaecol 1988; 159: 526–530.
40. Speth RC, Bumpus FM, Husain A. Identification of angiotensin II receptors in the rat ovary. Eur J Pharmacol 1986; 130: 351–452.
41. Husain A, Bumpus FM, DeSilva P, Speth RC. Localization of angiotensin II receptors in ovary follicles and the identification of angiotensin II in rat ovaries. Proc Natl Acad Sci USA 1987; 84: 2489–2494.
42. Speth RC, Husain A. Distribution of angiotensin-converting enzyme and angiotensin II-receptor binding sites in the rat ovary. Biol Reproduc 1988; 38: 695–702.
43. Grady EF, Sechi LA, Griffin CA, Schambelan M, Kalinyak JE. Expression of AT2 receptors in the developing rat fetus. J Clin Invest 1991; 88: 921–933.
44. Tsutsumi K, Stromberg C, Viswanathan M, Saavedra JM. Angiotensin-II receptor subtypes in fetal tissues of the rat: autoradiography, guanine nucleotide sensitivity, and association with phosphoinositide hydrolisis. Endocrinology 1991; 129: 1075–1082.
45. Pobiner BF, Northup JK, Bauer PH, Fraser ED, Garrison JC. Inhibitory GTP- binding regulatory protein G13 can couple angiotensin II receptors to inhibition of adenylyl cyclase in hepatocytes. Mol Pharmacol 1991; 40: 156–167.
46. Johnson MC, Aguilera G. Angiotensin-II receptor subtypes and coupling to signaling systems in cultured fetal fibroblasts. Endocrinology 1991; 129: 1266–1274.
47. Matsubara H, Kanasaki M, Murasawa S, Tsukaguchi Y, Nio Y, Inada M. Differential gene expression and regulation of angiotensin II receptor subtypes in rat cardiac fibroblasts and cardiomyocytes in culture. J Clin Invest 1994; 93: 1592–1601.
48. Johnson AR, Ashton J, Schulz WW, Erdšs EG. Neutral metalloendopeptidase in human lung tissue and cultured cells. Am Rev Respir Dis 1985; 132: 564–568.
49. Dostal DE, Rothblum KN, Chernin MI, Cooper GR, Baker KM. Intracardiac detection of angiotensin and renin: A localized renin-angiotensin system in neonatal rat heart. Am J Physiol 1992; 263: C838–C850.
50. Friedland J, Setton C, Silverstein E. Induction of angiotensin converting enzyme in human monocytes in culture. Biochem Biophys Res Comm 1978; 83(3): 843–849.
51. Krege JH, John SWM, Langenbach LL, et al. Male-female differences in fertility and blood pressure in ACE-deficient mice. Nature 1995; 375: 146–148.
52. Formigli L, Orlandini SZ, Benvenuti S, et al. In vitro structural and functional relationships between preosteoclastic and bone endothelial cells: A juxtacrine model for migration and adhesion of osteoclast precursors. J Cell Physiol 1995; 162: 199–212.

53. Takahashi N, Akatsu T, Udagawa N, et al. Osteoblastic cells are involved in osteoclast formation. Endocrinology 1988; 123(5): 2600–2602.
54. Moncada S, Palmer RMJ, Higgs EA. Nitric oxide: physiology, pathophysiology, and pharmacology. Pharmacol Rev 1991; 43(2): 109–142.
55. Lowick CWGM, Nibbering PH, van de Ruit M, Papapoulos SE. Inducible production of nitric oxide in osteoblast-like cells and in fetal mouse bone explants is associated with suppression of osteoclastic bone resorption. J Clin Invest 1994; 93: 1465–1472.
56. Palmer RMJ, Ferrige AG, Moncada S. Nitric oxide release accounts for the biological activity of endothelium derived relaxing factor. Nature 1987; 327: 524–526.
57. Fox SW, Chambers TJ, Chow JWM. Nitric oxide is an early mediator of the increase in bone formation by mechanical stimulation. Am J Physiol 1996; In press.
58. Norrdin RW, Jee WSS, High WB. Review: The role of prostaglandins in bone in vivo. Prostagl Leuk Ess Fatty Acids 1990; 41: 139–149.
59. Stimpel M, Jee WSS, Ma Y, Yamamoto N, Chen Y. Impact of antihypertensive therapy on postmenopausal osteoporosis: effects of the angiotensin converting enzyme inhibitor moexipril, 17β-estradiol and their combination on the ovariectomy-induced cancellous bone loss in young rats. J Hypertens 1995; 13: 1852–1856.

9 Effect of ACE-inhibition alone and in combination with 17-β-estradiol on the development of ovariectomy (postmenopausal)-induced bone loss in Sprague-Dawley-rats

Michael Stimpel and Webster S. S. Jee

Introduction

The rapid development of osteoporosis due to estrogen deficiency in women after menopause can be prevented by hormone (estrogen) replacement therapy (HRT) (1). Any concomitant drug therapy in postmenopausal women should therefore neither negatively influence the osteoprotective effects of HRT nor should it increase bone loss, when given alone. Though approximately 50% of the hypertensive population are postmenopausal females (for review see Ref. 2), little is known on whether long-term antihypertensive drug treatment affects the skeleton. Also, no data is available regarding the bone effects, when antihypertensive agents are coadministered with HRT.

The aim of the present study was to investigate the short- and long-term effects of the new ACE-inhibitor moexipril (3), 17β-estradiol, and a combination of both on the development of osteoporosis in the ovariectomized (ovx) Sprague-Dawley rat. This animal model is widely used for assessing preventive therapies against bone loss due to estrogen deficiency, since it has proved to excellently mimic the skeletal changes of postmenopausl osteoporosis in humans (4, 5, 6).

Materials and methods

One hundred nineteen 12-week-old virgin female Sprague-Dawley rats (Simonsen Laboratory, Inc., Gilroy, CA, U.S.A.) were acclimated to local vivarium, conditions, fed a commercial diet and provided with water ad libitum. Seven rats were sacrificed on day 0 as basal controls. The remaining rats were divided into sham-ovariectomy (sham-ovx) or ovariectomy (ovx) groups. Vehicle, moexipril 10 mg/kg/d alone orally, 17β-estradiol 10 μg/kg/d alone subcutaneously, or their combination were given in sham-ovx or ovx rats immediately after operation for 14 (short-term effects) or 56 (long-term effects) days. The study protocol is shown in Table 9.1.

Table 9.1: Study design.

Treatment group	No. of rats killed		
	Week 0 (age 3 months)	Week 2 (age 3.5 months)	Week 8 (age 5 months)
Sham-ovx + vehicle	7	7	7
Ovx + vehicle		7	7
Sham-ovx + moexipril		7	7
Ovx + moexipril		7	7
Sham-ovx + 17β-estradiol		7	7
Ovx + 17β-estradiol		7	7
Sham-ovx + moexipril + 17β-estradiol		7	7
Ovs + moexipril + 17β-estradiol		7	7

Ovx, ovariectomy. Treatment: oral vehicle; oral moexipril at 10 mg/kg per day; subcutaneous 17β-estradiol at 10 μg/kg per day. Treatment was continuous until week 8 in all groups.

All rats were double-fluorescent labeled with 5 mg/kg calcein. Powder moexipril hydrochloride was dissolved in deionized water at a dose of 10 mg/1 ml, and 17β-estradiol (Sigma Chemical Co., St. Louis, MO, U.S.A.) was dissolved in a vehicle of 95% corn oil and 5% benzyl alcohol at a dose of 10 μg/1 ml (7, 8).

A stereology computer program (KSS Computer Engineer, Magna, Utah, USA) was used for measurement. Static histomorphometric measurements of primary spongiosa (the area 0 to 1.5 mm distal from the growth plate metaphyseal junction) and both static and dynamic histomorphometric measurements of secondary spongiosa (the area 1.5−4.5 mm distal from the growth plate metaphyseal junction) of the proximal tibial metaphysis (PTM) were performed on 20 mm undecalcified frontal sections. Static and dynamic histomorphometric measurements of the distal tibia proximal to the tibia fibular junction were performed on 30 mm undecalcified cross sections (9, 10, 11).

Data are presented as means ± standard deviation. One-way analysis of variance (ANOVA) with the Fisher PLSD was used to determine the statistical difference between groups (12). Probability (P) less than 0.05 was considered significant.

Results

Longitudinal bone growth (LGR) of the proximal tibia

There was a decrease in LGR from 3 to 5 months of age (aging effect). Ovariectomy stimulated LGR for 2 weeks, but not for 8 weeks. Moexipril treatment had no effect in either sham-ovx or ovx rats. 17β-estradiol treatment decreased LGR in both sham-ovx and ovx rats at both treatment periods. And moexipril plus 17β-estradiol treatment showed the same changes as 17β-estradiol alone.

Primary spongiosa of the proximal tibial metaphysis

There were no significant changes between 3 and 5 months of age. Ovariectomy induced cancellous bone loss by reducing trabecular numbers. Moexipril treatment had no effect on either sham-ovx or ovx rats. However, 17β-estradiol treatment alone for 8 weeks increased trabecular bone area, number and thickness in both rat groups. The moexipril plus 17β-estradiol treatment showed the same responses as 17β-estradiol alone.

Secondary spongiosa of the proximal tibial metaphysis

There was an age-related decrease bone formation and resorption between 3- (baseline) and 5-month-old rats. Ovariectomy induced trabecular bone loss accompanied by loss in trabecular numbers, due to increased bone turnover with resorption exceeding formation. Moexipril treatment given for 2 and 8 weeks had no effect on either sham-ovx or ovx rats. The 17β-estradiol treatment for 2 weeks prevented ovx-induced trabecular bone loss and the treatment for 8 weeks added extra trabecular bone to sham-ovx rats, and prevented trabecular bone loss in ovx rats (for detailed data see Table 9.2). In both treatment periods, there was a decreased bone turnover associated with depression of bone resorption greater than bone formation. Co-treatment of moexipril and 17β-estradiol had the same effect on sham-ovx and ovx rats as 17β-estradiol treatment alone. Figure 9.1 shows histomorphometric changes in the proximal tibial metaphysis.

Tibial shaft

There were no differences among all groups in total tissue, cortical bone and marrow areas after 2 and 8 weeks of treatment (data not shown). However, there were decreases in all periosteal and endocortical surfaces bone formation parameters in both by 8 weeks with aging (i. e., between 3 and 5 months). The ovariectomy effects at 2 weeks were limited to an increase in the eroded perimeter, while at 8 weeks there were depressions in endocortical osteoid surface indices at the $p < 0.05$ level. Moexipril had no effect on either sham-ovx or

Table 9.2: Histomorphometric changes in secondary spongiosa of proximal tibial metaphysis after 56 days of treatment.

	Trabecular area (%)	Labeled perimeter (%)	Osteoid perimeter (%)	Eroded perimeter (%)	Mineral apposition rate (μm/day)	Bone formation rate/BV (%/year)	Bone formation rate/TV (%/year)	Activation frequency (cycles/year)
Basal	15.0 ± 3.6	2.2 ± 0.4	10.8 ± 3.1	4.8 ± 1.3	2.0 ± 0.2	56.4 ± 15.5	8.3 ± 2.5	6.8 ± 1.9
Sham-ovx controls	15.5 ± 1.6*†	1.9 ± 1.3	3.6 ± 1.7*	2.5 ± 0.9*	0.8 ± 0.2*	17.2 ± 11.6*	2.8 ± 1.8*	1.0 ± 0.7*
Ovx controls	5.4 ± 3.0*†	8.0 ± 3.8*†	14.7 ± 6.0†	3.4 ± 1.8	0.8 ± 0.2*	85.2 ± 39.7†	4.2 ± 2.3*	4.2 ± 2.3*
Ovx + moexipril	5.9 ± 1.6*†	6.6 ± 2.6*†	11.4 ± 3.8†	4.0 ± 1.5	0.8 ± 0.2*	66.0 ± 30.8	3.8 ± 1.9*	3.0 ± 1.2*
Ovx + 17β-estradiol	16.1 ± 4.9*†	0.5 ± 0.3*†‡	1.6 ± 0.6*‡	1.2 ± 0.6*‡	0.7 ± 0.2*	4.0 ± 3.4*‡	0.6 ± 0.5*†‡	0.7 ± 0.2*‡
Ovx + cotreatment	16.2 ± 2.5*†	0.4 ± 0.3*†‡	1.2 ± 0.6*‡	1.1 ± 0.6*†‡	0.7 ± 0.2*	3.1 ± 2.7*†‡	0.5 ± 0.5*†‡	0.3 ± 0.3*‡

Ovx, ovariectomy; Bone formation rate/BV (bone volume), bone area referent; Bone formation rate/TV (tissue volume), bone volume referent; $^{*}P < 0.05$, versus basal; $^{\dagger}P < 0.05$, versus sham-ovariectomy controls; $^{\ddagger}P < 0.05$, versus ovariectomy controls.

Table 9.3: Dynamic histomorphometric changes in tibial shaft after 56 days of treatment.

	Periosteal surface			Endosteal surface				
	Labeled perimeter (%)	Mineral apposition rate (μm/day)	Bone formation rate/BS (μm/day × 100)	Labeled perimeter (%)	Eroded perimeter (%)	Osteoid perimeter (%)	Mineral apposition rate (μm/day)	Bone formation rate/BS (μm/day × 100)
Basal	61.3 ± 7.1	1.7 ± 0.2	105.6 ± 19.8	49.1 ± 15.4	0.9 ± 0.4	21.8 ± 14.3	0.7 ± 0.1	35.9 ± 17.8
Sham-ovx controls	47.1 ± 11.2*	1.2 ± 0.4*	57.2 ± 18.0*	18.4 ± 4.3*	0.7 ± 0.5	0.4 ± 0.5*	0.2 ± 0.4*	4.0 ± 10.5*
Ovx controls	57.1 ± 11.9	1.0 ± 0.2*	56.3 ± 18.8*	21.1 ± 3.8*	0.5 ± 0.4	3.5 ± 3.6*†	0.1 ± 0.1*	1.1 ± 2.8*
Ovx + moexipril	62.3 ± 12.4	1.1 ± 0.2*	67.9 ± 19.4*	24.2 ± 5.1*	0.4 ± 0.3*	2.8 ± 1.4*†	0.2 ± 0.3*	5.7 ± 7.7*
Ovx + 17β-estradiol	7.9 ± 6.5*†‡	0.1 ± 0.3*†‡	2.1 ± 4.8*‡†	7.9 ± 4.1*†‡	0.2 ± 0.2*†	0.1 ± 0.4‡		
Ovx + cotreatment	15.1 ± 15.0*†‡	0.3 ± 0.3*†‡	9.0 ± 12.7*†‡	4.1 ± 2.9*†‡	0.3 ± 0.3*	0.8 ± 1.0*‡		

Ovx, ovariectomy; bone formation rate/BS (bone surface), bone surface referent. $^{*}P < 0.05$, versus basal; $^{\dagger}P < 0.05$, versus sham-ovariectomy controls; $^{\ddagger}P < 0.05$, versus ovariectomy controls.

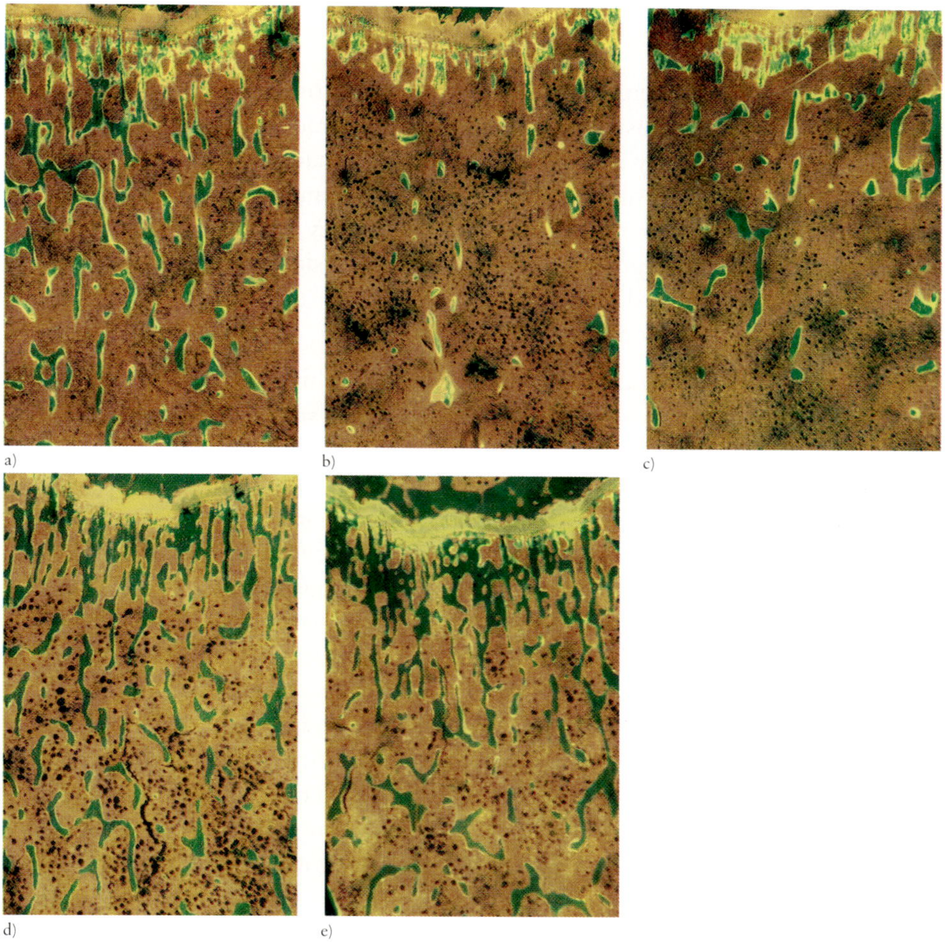

Figure 9.1 a–e: Microphotography of changes in the proximal tibial metaphysis in intact, ovariectomized and treated ovariectomized Sprague–Dawley rats. (a) A 5-month-old rat shows normal growth plate, normal trabecular bone mass, well connected trabecular (good network connection) and normal label distribution. (b) the effects of ovariectomy include a dramatic bone loss 8 weeks after the operation (at the age of 3 months) associated with increasing bone turnover. (c) Ovariectomy + moexipril treatment (8 weeks) shows no obvious difference from ovariectomy alone (Fig. 9.1 b). (d) Ovariectomy + 17β-estradiol treatment (8 weeks) increased the trabecular area in primary spongiosa and prevented ovariectomy-induced bone loss in secondary spongiosa by depressing bone turnover. (e) Ovariectomy and 17β-estradiol + moexipril (8 weeks) produced the same effects as 17β-estradiol alone (Fig. 9.1 d).

ovx rats. By 8 weeks, 17β-estradiol treatment decreased all periosteal bone formation indices as well as endocortical labeled perimeter compared with the respective controls. The 17β-estradiol treated rats possessed no double-fluorescent label. Co-treatment of 17β-estradiol plus moexipril showed the same changes as 17β-estradiol treatment alone (Table 9.3).

Discussion

The effects of antihypertensive therapy alone or in combination with hormone replacement on osteoporosis in postmenopausal women have not been studied so far. In the present study we investigated the pharmacological effects of short-term and long-term ACE-inhibition alone and in combination with 17β-estradiol on the bone turnover in the ovx Sprague-Dawley rat, a generally accepted animal model to mimic postmenopausal osteoporosis in humans sharing the same cause (i. e. estrogen deficiency) and mechanism (increase of bone turnover and resorption greater than formation) (4, 5, 6).

The rationale for investigating the effect of ACE inhibition on the bone turnover in estrogen-deficiency states is based on the following findings: Firstly, osteoclasts, the "driving force" for postmenopausal bone loss (13, 14), are in close proximity to the blood capillaries of the metaphyseal bone marrow. Secondly, osteoclasts have shown to be target cells for substances released by the endothelium of the bone microvasculature such as endothelin (ET-1) (15, 16), nitric oxide (17) or prostaglandins (18, 19, 20), suggesting that in addition to systemic hormonal regulation osteoclasts might also be locally regulated by endothelial products (16). – Since the endothelium has also been identified as both a target and a source of the renin angiotensin system (RAS) (21, 22), it was tempting to speculate whether the RAS might be involved in the regulation of the bone turnover. Theoretically, angiotensin II (Ang II) could influence the bone turnover in two ways: either indirectly by acting as a vasoconstrictor locally regulating the blood flow in the bone marrow capillaries or directly by acting as a "growth" hormone influencing the activation and/or proliferation of osteoclasts and/or osteoblasts. The latter speculation is supported by in vitro experiments having shown that osteoclasts cocultured with calvarial cells, or sedimented with contaminant bone cells were activated by Ang I (and Ang II) and inhibited by moexiprilat, suggesting that the RAS may play a role in the regulation of osteoclastic bone resorption (23).

Under in vivo conditions as in the present study, monotherapy of moexipril at the dosage given did not affect the skeleton. As expected, 17β-estradiol protected the rats against trabecular bone loss, which typically occurs in estrogen deficiency states such as postmenopausal osteoporosis (23). The osteoprotective effects of 17β-estradiol were not influenced in either direction when moexipril was coadministered neither on a short-term nor on a long-term basis.

From these findings one might follow that the RAS and its pharmacological inhibition are not of (patho)physiological importance for the regulation of the bone turnover under in vivo conditions in estrogen deficiency states such as the physiological or artificial postmenopause.

However, this study has a number of limitations: Firstly, only one dosage has been used in this trial. Secondly, due to methodologic reasons it was not possible to either investigate the impact of ACE-inhibition on blood flow in the microvasculature of the bone marrow or the penetration of moexipril into the bone, the latter being a prerequisite for any potential effects on local tissue ACE. Thirdly, since bone turnover was the primary endpoint in this study, we investigated the moexipril effects in the ovx Sprague-Dawley rat. This was a compromise since a suitable animal model concomitantly mimicing both human postmenopausal osteoporosis and hypertension is not available so far.

In summary, we follow that short-term and long-term ACE-inhibition by moexipril alone or in combination with hormone replacement therapy does not affect the skeleton in ovx Sprague-Dawley rats. The clinical relevance of these findings has to be confirmed.

Acknowledgement

Originally published in Journal of Hypertension 1995, Volume 13 and reprinted with permission of the publisher Rapid Science Publishers, 2–6, Boundary Row, London, SE1 8HN, UK. Tel.: (+44) 171 8650198 Fax: (+44) 171 9286293.

References

1. Horowitz MC. Cytokines and estrogen in bone: anti-osteoporotic effects. Science 1993; 260: 626
2. Safar M, Stimpel M, Zanchetti A (eds.): Hypertension in Postmenopausal Women. Berlin Heidelberg New York: Springer-Verlag, 1994, 1–87.
3. Stimpel M. Moexipril. In Messerli FH (ed.): Cardiovascular Drug Therapy 2nd ed. Philadelphia: WB Saunders, 1996: 813–816.
4. Wronski TJ Walsh CC, Ignaszewski LS. Histologic evidence for osteopenia and increased bone turnover in ovariectomized rats. Bone 1986; 7: 119–123.
5. Yamazaki I, Yamaguchi H. Characteristics of an ovariectomized rat model. J Bone Min Res 1989; 4(1): 13–22.
6. Kalu DN, Chung-Ching L, Hardin RR, Hollis BW. The aged rat model of ovarian hormone deficiency bone loss. Endocrinology 1989; 124: 7–16.
7. Wronski TJ, Cintron M, Dogherty AL, Dann LM. Estrogen treatment prevents osteopenia and depresses bone turnover in ovariectomized rats. Endocrinology 1988; 123: 681–686.
8. Wronski TJ, Yen CF, Scott KS. Estrogen and diphosphonate treatment provide long-term protection against osteopenia in ovariectomized rats. J Bone Min Res 1991; 6: 387–394.
9. Parfitt AM, Drezner MK, Glorieux FH, Kanis JA, Malluche H, Meunier PJ, Ott SM, Recker RR. Bone histomorphometry: Standardization of nomenclature, symbols, and units. J Bone Min Res 1987; 2: 595–610.
10. Jee WSS, Mori S, Li XJ, Chan S. Prostaglandin E_2 enhances cortical bone mass and activates intracortical bone remodeling in intact and ovariectomized female rats. Bone 1990; 11: 253–266.
11. Mori S, Jee WSS, Li SJ. Production of new trabecular bone in osteopenic ovariectomized rats by prostaglandin E_2. Calcif Tissue Int 1992; 50: 80–87.

12. Neter J, Wasserman W, Whitmore GA. Applied Statistics. Allyn and Bacon, Boston 1982, pp. 544–572.
13. Partitt AM. Bone-forming cells in clinical conditions. In Hall BK (ed.): The osteoblast and osteocyte. Vol 1 of Bone. Boca Raton, Fla: Telford Press/CRC Press, 1990: 351–429.
14. Eriksen EF, Hodgson SF, Eastell R, Cedel SL, O'Fallon WM, Riggs BL: Cancellous bone remodeling in type 1 (postmenopausal) osteoporosis: quantitative assessment of rates of formation, resorption, and bone loss at tissue and cellular levels. J Bone Min Res 1990; 5: 311–319.
15. Alam ASMT, Gallagher A, Shankar V, Ghatei MA, Datta HK, Huang CLH. Endothelin inhibits osteoclastic bone resportion by a direct effect on cell motility: implications for the vascular control of bone resorption. Endocrinology 1992; 130: 3617–3624.
16. Sasaki T, Hong MH. Localization of Endothelin-1 in the Osteoclast. J Electron Microsc 1993; 4: 193–196
17. MacIntyre I, Zaidi M, Alam ASMT, Datta HK, Moonga BS, Lidbury P, et al. Osteoclastic inhibiton: an action of mitric oxide not mediated by cyclic GMP. Proc Natl Acad Sci USA 1991; 88: 2936–2940.
18. Jee WSS, Mori S, Li XJ, Chan S. Prostaglandin E_2 enhances cortical bone mass and activates intracortical bone remodeling in intact and ovariectomized female rats. Bone 1990; 11: 253–266.
19. Mori S, Jee WSS, Li XJ, Chan S, Kimmel DB. Effects of prostaglandin E_2 on production of new cancellous bone in the axial skeleton of ovariectomized rats. Bone 1990; 11: 103–113.
20. Jee WSS, Ke HZ, Li XJ. Long-term anabolic effect of prostaglandin E_2 on tibial diaphyseal bone in male rats. Bone and Mineral 1991; 15: 33–55.
21. Campbell DJ. Tissue renin-angiotensin system: sites of angiotensin formation. J Cardiovasc Pharmacol 1987; 10(suppl 7): S1–S8.
22. Ganten D, Hermann K, Unger T, Lang RE. The tissue renin-angiotensin systems: focus on brain angiotensins, adrenal gland, and arterial wall. Clin Exp Hypertens 1983; 5: 1099–1118.
23. Hatton R, Stimpel M, Chambers TJ. Angiotensin II is generated from angiotensin I by bone cells and stimulates osteoclastic bone resorption in vitro. J Endocrinol, in press.
24. Manolagas SC, Jilka RL. Bone marrow, cytokines, and bone remodeling. N Eng J Med 1995; 332: 305–311.

10 Sex specific mechanisms of cardiovascular disease

Theo Pelzer and Ludwig Neyses

Introduction

Estrogens have long been known to determine many of the sex specific differences in normal individuals and in disease. As far as cardiovascular diseases are concerned, most studies have focused on men because of their higher incidence of myocardial infarction and stroke. Therefore, the natural course and the efficiency of interventions are largely unknown for the female population. It is only very recently that the dramatic changes in the role of women in modern societies have lead to the perception that different diagnostic and therapeutic strategies are required in female versus male individuals. This is all the more surprising since gender specific differences in the incidence of cardiovascular disease have long been known (1). Pre-menopausal women have a significantly lower risk than men to develop coronary heart disease. In contrast, after menopause this risk increases rapidly to levels that are largely equal to males. There are only few studies which have investigated the effects of estrogen replacement therapy in heart disease, but it has been claimed that estrogen substitution leads to a 30–50% decrease in cardiovascular mortality compared to untreated postmenopausal women (2). Therefore, estrogens may represent a very powerful tool for the treatment of cardiovascular disease. However the widespread therapeutic application of estrogens is currently limited by the fact that very little is known about the mechanisms of estrogen action in normal and pathological cardiovascular tissues.

It is the aim of this short review to give an oversight of what is known about the biological effects of estrogens and to point out where future research should be directed.

General principles of estrogen action

Grossly, the mechanisms of estrogen action may be divided into two parts: One is the classical genomic effect known from other steroid hormones. However, estrogens also have a host of non-genomic effects which are only beginning to be characterized and will thus be discussed only shortly in this review because of our lack of knowledge.

Adrenal steroids, vitamin D, and estrogens comprise the steroid hormone family. They all act by a basically similar mechanism. Unlike most other hormones, their biological effects are not mediated by cell surface receptors. Instead they pass the cell membrane and bind highly specific to receptors located in the cytoplasm, which upon hormone binding translocates into the nucleus. They then bind to DNA as a hormone-receptor complex which activates transcription of specific genes. Whereas adrenal steroids, vitamin D and thyroid hormone receptors dimerize with other proteins, the DNA binding of the estrogen receptor occurs almost exclusively as a homodimer. DNA binding of the estrogen receptor occurs at a short cis-acting DNA sequence in the regulatory region (promoter) of estrogen responsive genes which share the highly conserved base sequence (5′ AGGTCA 3′). Typically two of these half-sites are arranged in head to tail orientation (as palindromes), separated by three variable base pairs. This arrangement is called an estrogen responsive element (ERE, 3). It has recently become evident that ERE half sites as direct repeats or single elements can also mediate genomic estrogen effects (4). The basic mechanisms of estrogen receptor mediated gene expression are outlined in Figure 10.1.

The estrogen receptor was one of the few human genes that had been cloned as early as 1985 (5). Meanwhile the modular structure of the estrogen receptor

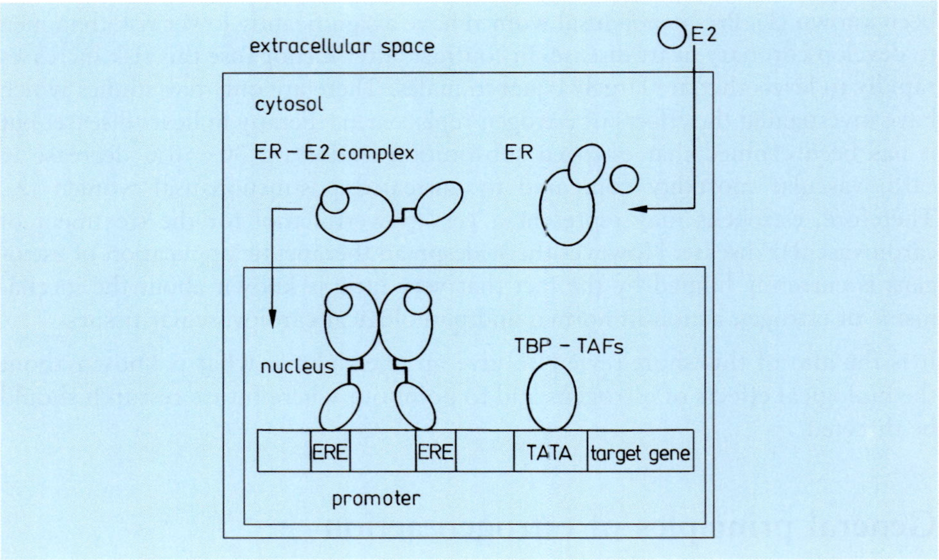

Figure 10.1: The estrogen receptor (ER) functions as a ligand dependent transcription factor. Extracellular estrogen (E2) passes the cell membrane probably due to its lipophilic properties. The estrogen receptor undergoes a conformational change upon ligand binding. The receptor-ligand complex (ER-E2 complex) tranclocates into the nucleus. Formation of ER homodimers facilitates cooperative DNA binding to estrogen response elements (ERE) in the promoter region of estrogen responsive target genes. Transcriptional activation or repression of the promoter is mediated by direct or indirect interactions (including additional factors) with the basal transcription machinery represented by the TATA-box binding protein (TBP) and associated factors (TAFs).

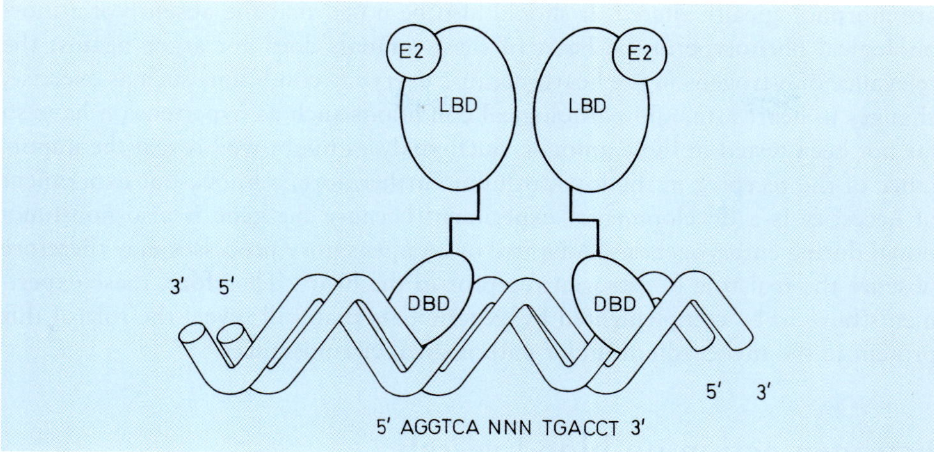

Figure 10.2: The estrogen receptor contains several different functional domains. The diagram illustrates the DNA binding of an estrogen receptor homodimer to a canonical estrogen response element (ERE). The ERE is composed of two half sites in head to tail orientation which are separated by three random base pairs. Estrogen (E2) binding of the receptor occurs at the ligand binding domain (LBD). Each receptor monomer contacts an ERE half site by its DNA binding domain (DBD).

has been studied extensively. Figure 10.2 gives a rough picture of the domain organization of the estrogen receptor. A DNA-binding domain makes contact with the DNA at the ERE sequence, whereas the ligand-binding domain serves as the part of the molecule which binds estrogens with high affinity and specificity. A considerable number of other regulatory regions of the estrogen receptor have been identified by analysis of estrogen receptor mutants. Among these are transcriptional activation domains, dimerization surfaces, phosphorylation sites and regions that contact additional transcription factors (6, 7). These aspects are not further discussed here because of the very limited knowledge of the role of these processes in the heart. It should be noted however, that there are instances where DNA binding of the estrogen receptor is dispensable for the transcriptional regulation of target genes in which the estrogen receptor regulates transcriptional activity by interaction with other transcription factors. This has been paradigmatically shown by binding of an estrogen receptor mutant lacking the DNA binding domain to the AP-1 site, which binds the FOS/JUN complex (8). Furthermore, there may be elements other than the classical "estrogen response element" which the estrogen receptor binds to (probably indirectly), such as a AT-rich sequence in the brain creatine kinase promoter (9).

Of particular interest is the recent description of a "knock-out" mutation for the estrogen receptor in the mouse system (10). These mice are viable but infertile (this is true for both sexes). It is of note that infertility in males had been unexpected. The testes of these animals are small and the seminiferous tubules are morphologically altered. It should also be noted that the absence of a morphological phenotype in the heart of these animals does not argue against the relevance of estrogens in the heart, because everyday conditions such as exercise, changes in heart rate, and pathological conditions such as hypertension have so far not been tested in these animals. Such analyses might well reveal the importance of the receptor in the myocardium. Furthermore, a knock-out experiment of necessity is a developmental experiment because the gene is also non-functional during embryogenesis. Adaptive or compensatory processes may therefore obscure the real role of estrogen receptor in the heart. Therefore, these experiments have to be complemented by experiments that will reveal the role of this protein in the myocardium under pathological circumstances.

Estrogen action on blood vessels

As early as 1884 MacKenzie described increased blood flow in mucosal membranes during the menstrual cycle and pregnancy (11). Estrogens have since been shown to acutely dilate arterial vessels, including coronary arteries

Table 10.1: Potential target genes for estrogen regulation*.

Target gene	Reference #
angiotensin-I converting enzyme	21, 22
c-fos	23, 24
c-myc	25
c-jun	24
prostacyclin synthase	36
prostaglandin cyclooxygenase	36
α-myosin heavy chain	26, 17
β-myosin heavy chain	26, 17
egr-1	24
estrogen receptor	27
insulin-like-growth-factor-1	28
elastin	29
collagen	29
connexin 43	30
heat shock protein 27	31, 32
nitric oxide synthase isoform 1	33
nitric oxide synthase isoform 2	34, 35
nitric oxide synthase isoform 3	15

* Overview of candidate genes, which are likely but not yet proven to be transcriptionally regulated by the estrogen receptor. These genes are relevant to the cardiovascular system and have either been shown to be regulated by estrogen in non-cardiac tissues or they contain estrogen response elements in their regulatory regions. Numbering refers to references.

within 5–10 minutes (12). This rapid onset strongly suggests a non-genomic mechanism because it is unlikely to require new protein synthesis. In addition, there is strong evidence for transcriptional regulation of gene expression in the vasculature by 17β-estradiol. This has been suggested first by binding of radioactive estradiol to aortic tissue. Meanwhile, transcriptional regulation of the progesterone receptor, which is well known to be upregulated by estrogen in many tissues (13), has been shown convincingly in vascular tissues. Recent results have also demonstrated that human saphenous vein smooth muscle cells contain functional estrogen receptors (14). Similar approaches showed up-regulation of nitric oxide synthase (eNOS) by estrogen in cultured human endothelial cells (15). The exact mechanism of estrogen interaction with cell cycle regulatory factors, by which they either promote (i. e. breast cancer cells) or repress cell proliferation (i. e. vascular fibroblasts), remain to be defined. A major challenge for future work lies in defining the physiological target genes for estrogen in the vasculature (see Table 10.1 for a speculative list of candidate genes).

Estrogen action on the myocardium

Very little is known about this question. In early studies almost 20 years ago uptake of radioactive labeled estrogen into the myocardium had been shown. This line of investigation was however abandoned, because the methodology to analyze molecular mechanisms was not available until recently. Studies by Morano et al. have shown that testosterone treatment increases the amount of the V3 isoform of the myosin heavy chain pattern in the myocardium of spontaneously hypertensive rats (16). This results can be interpreted as showing that sex specific mechanisms in cardiac hypertrophy do exist. Furthermore, in whole animal experiments it has been shown that estradiol influences the myosin heavy chain isoform pattern in female rats (17).

Our own recent approach has been to investigate the mechanisms of estrogen action on the myocardium itself. Immunofluorescence and Western blot studies showed the presence of estrogen receptors in isolated rat neonatal myocardial cells. These estrogen receptors are functional as demonstrated by the fact that they were able to induce transcription from a minigene composed of a triple estrogen responsive element coupled to a minimal promoter and the cDNA for luciferase (18). Future studies are now directed towards defining the target genes of the estrogen receptor in the myocardium.

Non-genomic effects of estrogens in the cardiovascular system

A host of steroid hormone effects have been described which are independent of nuclear hormone receptors. The operational definition of a non-genomic effect is that it does not require de-novo protein synthesis and more practically by its very rapid onset of action (seconds to minutes after application of the hormone). In contrast, genomic effects require time for the expression of mRNA and protein and thus are characterized by a delayed onset, which may need several hours after application of hormone. Very little is known about the molecules that interact with estrogens besides the estrogen receptor. A calcium antagonistic effect of estrogen has been described in guinea pig cardiac myocytes at high estrogen concentrations (19). More convincing are data that show interaction of estrogens with potassium activated calcium channels at physiological hormone levels (20). The problem with many of these studies is that the concentrations of estrogen employed in these experiments are well above the physiological range which is 0.1 nM before puberty, after menopause and in male individuals. During the follicular phase of the menstrual cycle, the maximum serum estrogen concentration is about 0.6 nM, about 1–10 nM are attained during pregnancy. In contrast to these non-genomic effects, our own studies have employed estrogen at physiological concentrations (18).

Future outlook

Understandably, there is great interest in potential applications of estrogen therapy in cardiac disease. Many estrogen derivatives are currently being used for the treatment of diseases such as osteoporosis and are already on the market. However extensive in-vitro and in-vivo animal studies on the beneficial effects of estrogens in the myocardium are required before estrogen treatment could become clinical practice. Work in this direction is ongoing in our laboratory.

Acknowledgements

The authors acknowledge the extensive help by Mrs. S. Oberdorf-Maass and the members of the laboratory as well as Dr. C. Grohé, Medical Policlinic, University of Bonn.

References

1. Glendy RE, Levine SA, White PD. Coronary disease in youth: comparison of 100 patients under 40 with 300 persons past 80. JAMA 1937; 109: 1775–1781.
2. Stampfer MJ, Colditz GA, Willett WC, Manson JE, Rosner B, Speizer FE, Hennekens CH. Postmenopausal estrogen therapy and cardiovascular disease. N Engl J Med 1991; 325: 756–762.
3. Klein-Hitpass L, Schorpp M, Wagner W, Ryffel GU. An estrogen responsive element derived from the 5′ flanking region of the xenopus vitellogenin A12 gene functions in transfected human cells. Cell 1986; 46: 1053–1061.
4. Kato S, Sasaki H, Suzawa M, Masushige S, Tora L, Chambon P, Gronemeyer H. Widely spaced, directly repeated PuGGTCA elements act as promiscuous enhancers for different classes of nuclear receptors. Mol Cell Biol 1995; 15: 5858–5867.
5. Walter P, Green S, Krust A, Bornert JM, Jeltsch JM, Staub A, Jensen E, Scrace G, Waterfield M, Chambon P. Cloning of the human estrogen receptor cDNA. Proc Natl Acad Sci USA 1985; 82: 7889–7893.
6. Kumar V, Green S, Staub A, Chambon P. Localisation of the estradiol-binding and putative DNA-binding domains of the human estrogen receptor. EMBO J 1986; 5: 2231–2236.
7. Migliaccio A, Di Domenico M, Green S, de Falco A, Kajtaniac EL, Blasi F, Chambon P, Auricchio F. Phosphorylation on tyrosine of in vitro synthezised human estrogen receptor activates its hormone binding. Mol Endocrinol 1989; 3: 1061–1069.
8. Gaub MP, Bellard M, Scheuer I, Chambon P, Sassone-Corsi P. Activation of the ovalbumin gene by the estrogen receptor involves the fos-jun complex. Cell 1990; 63: 1267–1276.
9. Sukovich DA, Mukherjee R, Benfield PA. A novel, cell-type-specific mechanism for estrogen receptor mediated gene activation in the absence of an estrogen- responsive element. Mol Cell Biol 1994; 14: 7134–7143.
10. Lubahn DB, Moyer JS, Golding TS, Couse JF, Korach KS, Smithies O. Alteration of reproductive function but not prenatal sexual development after insertional disruption of the mouse estrogen receptor gene. Proc Natl Acad Sci USA 1993; 90: 11162–11166.
11. MacKenzie J. Irritation of the sexual apparatus. Am J Med Sci 1884; 87: 360.
12. Silva de Sa MF, Meirelles RS. Vasodilatation effect of estrogen on the human umbilical artery. Gynecol Invest 1977; 8: 307.
13. Horwitz KB, Horwitz LD. Canine vascular tissues are targets for androgens, estrogens, progestins and glucocorticoids. J Clin Invest 1982; 69: 750.
14. Karas RH, Patterson BL, Mendelsohn ME. Human vascular smooth muscle cells contain functional estrogen receptor. Circulation 1994; 98: 1943–1950.
15. Hishikawa K, Nakaki K, Marumo T, Suzuki H, Kato R, Saruta T. Up-regulation of nitric oxide synthase by estradiol in human aortic endothelial cells. FEBS Lett 1995; 360: 291–293.
16. Morano I, Gerstner J, Rüegg JC, Ganten U. Regulation of myosin heavy chain expression in the hearts of hypertensive rats by testosterone. Circ Res 1990; 66: 1585–1590.
17. Malhotra A, Buttrick P, Scheuer J. Effects of sex hormones on development of physiological and pathological cardiac hypertrophy in male and female rats. Am J Physiol 1990; 259: H866–H871.
18. Grohe C, Kahlert S, Löbbert K, Stimpel M, Karas RH, Vetter H, Neyses L. Cardiac myocytes and fibroblasts contain functional estrogen receptors. Circulation 1994; 90: Suppl. I 538.
19. Jiang C, Poole-Wilson PA, Sarrel PM, Mochizuki S, Collins P, McLeod KT. Effect of 17β-estradiol on concentration, Ca2+ current and intracellular free Ca2+ in guinea-pig isolated cardiac myocytes. Br J Pharmacol 1992; 106: 739–745.
20. White RE, Darkow DJ, Falvo Lang JL. Estrogen relaxes coronary arteries by opening BkCa channels through a cGMP-dependent mechanism. Circ Res 1995; 77: 936–942.

21. Proudler AJ, Ahmed Al H, Crook D, Fogelman I, Rymer JM, Stevenson JC. Hormone replacement therapy and serum angiotensin-converting-enzyme activity in post-menopausal women. Lancet 1995; 346: 89–90.
22. Testut P, Soubrier F, Corvol P, Hubert C. Functional analysis of the human somatic angiotensin-I converting enzyme gene promoter. Biochem J 1993; 293: 843–848.
23. Weisz A, Rosales R. Identification of an estrogen response element upstream of the human c-fos gene that binds the estrogen receptor and the AP-1 transcription factor. Nucleic Acids Res 1990; 18: 5097–5106.
24. Cicatiello L, Sica V, Bresciani F, Weisz A. Identification of a specific pattern of "immediate-early" gene activation induced by estrogen during mitogenic stimulation of rat uterine cells. Receptor 1993; 3: 17–30.
25. Dubik D, Dembinski TC, Shiu RPC. Stimulation of the c-myc oncogene expression associated with estrogen-induced proliferation of human breast cancer cells. Cancer Res 1987; 47: 6517–6521.
26. Morano I, Gagelmann M, Arner A, Ganten U, Rüegg JC. Myosin isoenzymes of vascular smooth and cardiac muscle in the spontaneously hypertensive and normotensive male and female rat: a comparative study. Circ Res 1986; 59: 456–462.
27. Katzenellenbogen BS, Nardulli AM, Read LD. Estrogen regulation of proliferation and hormonal modulation of estrogen and progesterone receptor biosynthesis and degradation in target cells. Prog Clin Biol Res 1990; 322: 201–211.
28. Michels KM, Lee WH, Seltzer A, Saavedra JM, Bondy CA. Up-regulation of pituitary [125] insulin-like growth factor-I (IGF-I) binding and IGF-I binding protein-2 and IGF-I gene expression by estrogen. Endocrinology 1993; 132: 23–29.
29. Cembran J, Lillo M, Val J, Mardones J. Influence of sex difference and hormones on elastin and collagen in aorta of chickens. Circ Res 1960; 8: 527.
30. Yu W, Dahl G, Werner R. The connexin-43 gene is responsive to estrogen. Proc R Soc Lond 1994; 255: 125–132.
31. Fuqua SAW, Blum-Saringos M, McGuire WL. Induction of the estrogen-regulated "24K" protein by heat shock. Cancer Res 1984; 49: 4126.
32. Mendelsohn ME, Zhu Y, O'Neill S. The 29-kDa proteins phosphorylated in thrombin-activated platelets are forms of the estrogen receptor-related 27 kDa heat shock protein. Proc Natl Acad Sci USA 1991; 88: 11212–11216.
33. Weiner C, Lizasoain I, Baylis SA, Knowles RG, Charles IG, Moncada S. Induction of calcium-dependent nitric oxide synthases by sex hormones. Proc Natl Acad Sci 1994; 91: 5212–5216.
34. Xie QW, Cho H, Calaycay J, Mumford R, Swiderek KM, Lee TB, Ding A, Troso T, Nathan C. Cloning and characterization of inducible nitric oxide synthase from mouse macrophage. Science 1992; 256: 225–228.
35. Xie QW, Whisnant R, Nathan C. Promoter of the mouse gene encoding calcium- independent nitric oxide synthase confers inducibility by interferon-gamma and bacterial lipopolysaccharides. J Exp Med 1993; 177: 1779–1784.
36. Chang WC, Nakao J, Orimo H, Murota SI. Stimulation of prostaglandin cyclooxygenase and prostacyclin synthase activities by estradiol in rat aortic smooth muscle cells. Biochem Biophys Acta 1980; 620: 472.

11 Arterial compliance in hypertension

Cristina Giannattasio, Monica Failla,
Maria Luisa Stella, Arduino A. Mangoni,
Stefano Carugo, Giuseppe Mancia

Introduction

Large and middle-size conduit arteries distend when blood is ejected from the left ventricle, thereby 1) limiting an excessive increase in systolic blood pressure and 2) providing, by recoiling, continuous rather than intermittent blood flow to the heart and all other organs (1). The major functions of these arteries are therefore compliance and distensibility to the inside pressure. This paper will describe data obtained by our group and others on the alterations of arterial compliance in hypertension and their reversal by treatment. This will be preceded by a brief section on technical problems in measuring compliance and followed by a resumè of the increasing evidence on arterial compliance alterations in cardiovascular as well as in non-cardiovascular diseases.

Methods for measuring arterial compliance

Studying arterial compliance in man has always been difficult, because all methods employed have shown major limitations. Methods for measuring compliance based on mathematical models, for example, have been characterized by the need for the models to limit the complexity of the factors involved in compliance determination, leading to use of oversimplified formulae. Measurements of compliance by direct assessment of arterial pressure and volume (the two variables from which compliance is derived), have, on the other hand, often turned out to be inaccurate, invasive and mostly limited to few accessible arteries.

Few years ago a technique was described that allows radial artery diameter to be continuously measured by ultrasonography, together with continuous non-invasive blood pressure measurements from an ipsilateral finger (2). Following extensive testing in three different laboratories (Lausanne, Paris and Milan), the technique was shown to possess a high discriminating power for tracking changes of arterial diameter and blood pressure over time (≤ 150 µm and ≤ 2 mmHg) (2, 3). It was also shown that both diameter and blood pressure measurements were reproducible (4) and that the diameter-pressure curves that were obtained were superimposable to those obtained when blood pressure was measured intra-arterially from the radial artery level, i. e. in the ideal condition in which both volume and pressure are derived from the same site (5). The stage was thus set for assessing arterial compliance more dynamically than ever done before, i. e. to derive its values by application of the Langewouters formula (6) as well as the distensibility values derived by dividing compliance for diameter over the entire diasto-systolic pressure range. This proved to be a crucial step forward, because compliance (and distensibility) values showed a steep curvilinear decrease with a blood pressure increase from diastole to systole. That is, compliance (and distensibility) showed a non-linear relationship with physiological blood pressure alterations which make compliance-pressure curves essential for describing their changes in different circumstances and diseases.

Hypertension and radial artery compliance

A time-honoured concept maintains that hypertension is characterized by a reduction of arterial compliance (7). Dynamic assessment of radial artery compliance by the method described above, however, has provided evidence that this is not invariably the case, because in middle age subjects with mild or moderate hypertension, compliance values were displaced upward over the entire diasto-systolic pressure range, compared to the values seen in normotensive control subjects (Figure 11.1) (8).

The reasons for this increase in compliance are unknown, but recent data allow some hypotheses to be made. One, in middle-age hypertensive subjects radial artery wall thickness (measured through the same device by which diameter is measured) (9) is increased (Figure 11.2) presumably because of an initial wall hypertrophy due to smooth muscle growth (10). Two, smooth muscle has a lower elastic modulus than connective tissue and its distensibility can be further increased if contraction is prevented by the intra-arterial infusion of a vasorelaxing agent, such as papaverine (Figure 11.3) (5). And three, smooth muscle relaxation can be induced, among other mechanisms, by endothelial relaxing factors. Although a number of studies reports that in hypertensive man secretion of these factors is impaired, there is also evidence that in the forearm of mild hypertensive patients no substantial reduction of the influence of the endothelial relaxing factor may occur (11). Indeed in hypertension the actual secretion of this factor may be increased because of an increase in endothelial shear stress (12). It can thus be speculated that in hypertension an increased smooth muscle growth in the arterial wall combines with a reduced smooth muscle contraction to largely maintain or increase middle-size conduit artery compliance (Figure 11.2).

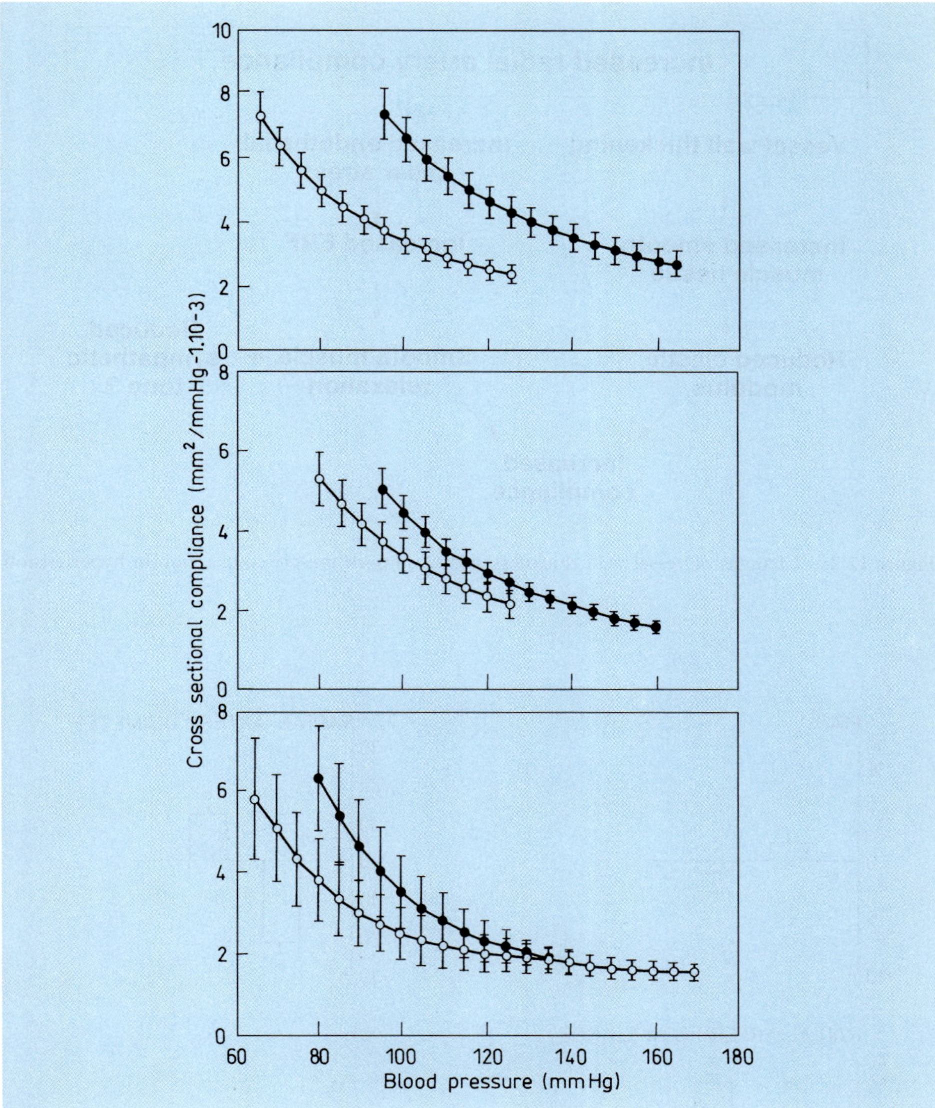

Figure 11.1: Cross sectional compliance/blood pressure curves in control subjects (open circles) and in mild hypertensive patients (closed circles), obtained in three different laboratories (Lausanne, Paris, Milan). Data from reference 8.

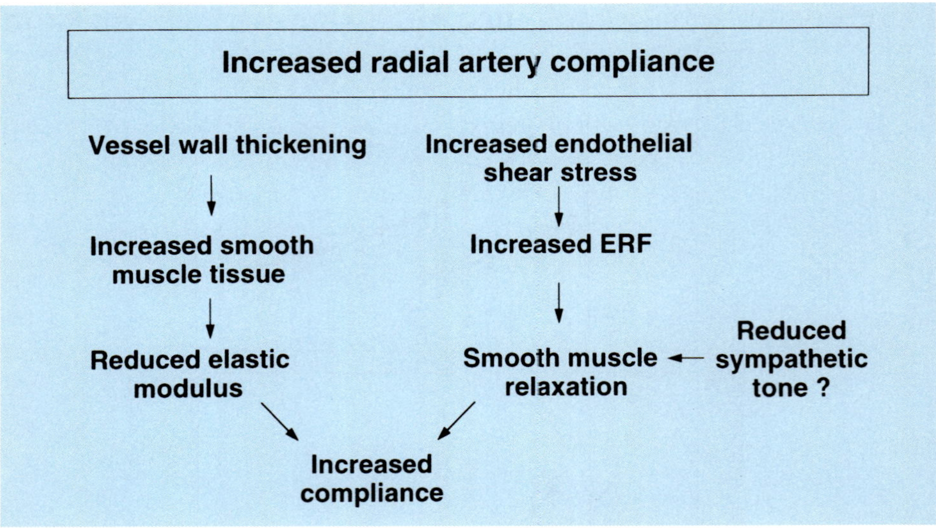

Figure 11.2: Changes of vessel wall thickness and of smooth muscle contraction in hypertension.

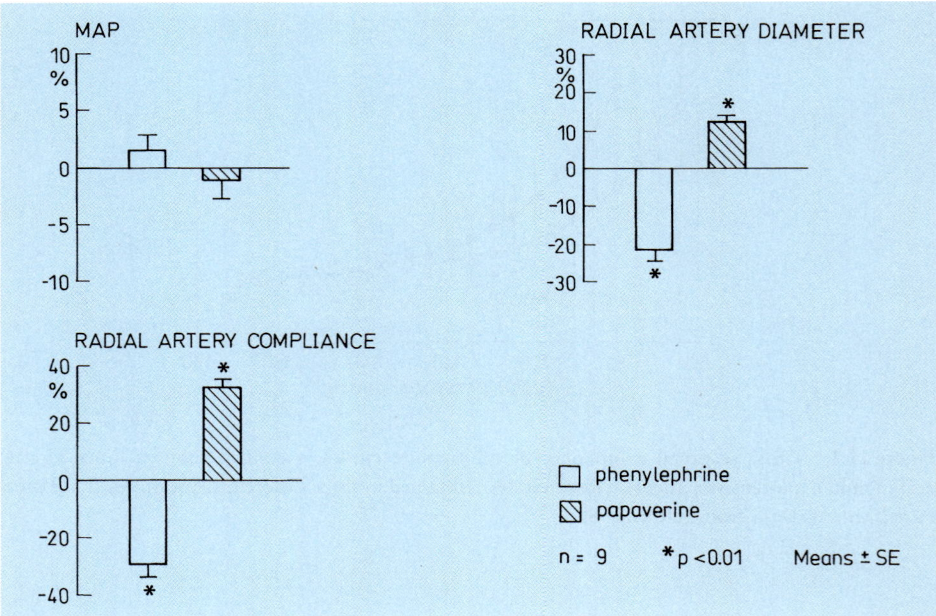

Figure 11.3: Changes in mean arterial blood pressure (MAP), radial artery diameter and compliance after local infusion of phenylephrine or papaverine. Data from reference 5.

Heterogeneity of compliance alterations in hypertension

In a number of old mild or moderate hypertensive subjects, radial artery compliance was assessed together with carotid artery compliance, using a sonographic approach to track continuous changes in common carotid diameter and calculating compliance values through the Reneman formula (13). Although lack of "in situ" blood pressure measurements prevented collection of "dynamic" compliance values, the data left no

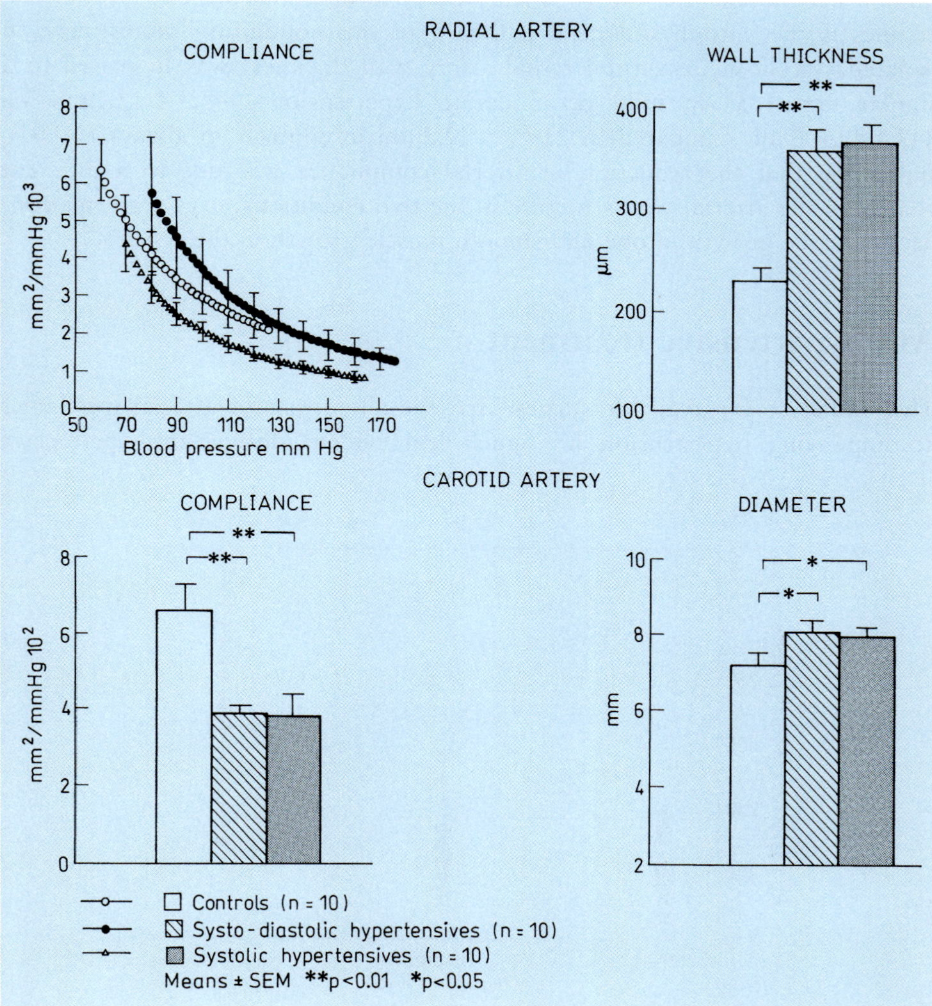

Figure 11.4: Line graphs show compliance/blood pressure curves of radial artery in control, systo-diastolic hypertensive and systolic hypertensive subjects. Histograms show radial artery wall thickness, carotid artery compliance and diameter in the three groups. Data from reference 14.

doubt that carotid artery compliance was reduced. The reduction was even more marked when age-matched subjects with an isolated systolic hypertension were considered and indeed in these subjects not only carotid but also radial artery compliance was less than in control individuals, at variance from the radial artery compliance data in mild or moderate hypertensives (Figure 11.4) (14).

Thus, mild or moderate hypertension is characterized by heterogeneous changes in compliance across the arterial tree. In isolated systolic hypertension, however, compliance is uniformly and markedly reduced in both large elastic and middle-size muscle arteries, which confirms that an impairment of arterial mechanics is the patophysiological hallmark of this condition. Interestingly, in isolated systolic hypertension radial artery wall thickness was increased to a similar extent as in mild or moderate hypertension (343.3 ± 12.1 μm vs. 343.1 ± 24.6 μm compared to 219.8 ± 12.2 μm in controls, p always < 0.01), suggesting that the reduction in arterial compliance was due to a different change in the arterial wall structure in the two conditions, e. g. a greater connective tissue growth in one and smooth muscle growth in the other.

Antihypertensive treatment

The studies so far available suggest that the alterations of arterial mechanics accompanying hypertension are much less evident during antihypertensive

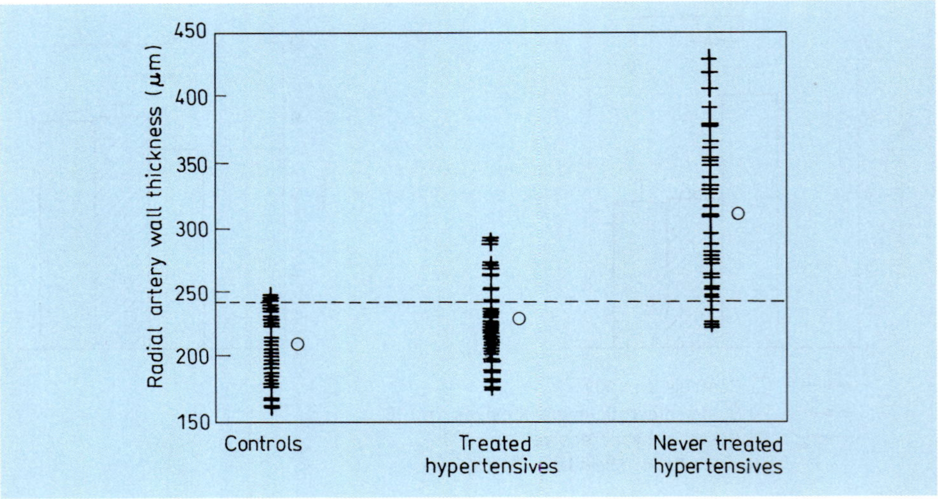

Figure 11.5: Individual data of radial artery wall thickness in normal subjects, in well-treated, and in never-treated hypertensive patients. Dashed line indicates the 95th percentile of normal values. Data from reference 16.

treatment. In mild or moderate hypertension, for example, the increase in radial artery compliance was shown to disappear after daily administration of lacidipine (15) or quinapril (Trazzi, Giannattasio and Mancia, unpublished observations). Furthermore, treated hypertensive patients were reported to have a radial artery wall thickness (and wall-to-lumen ratio) much less than that of untreated hypertensive patients and only slightly greater than that of normotensive control individuals (Figure 11.5) (16). Finally, in isolated systolic hypertension both the increased radial artery wall thickness and the reduced carotid artery compliance were found to be significantly reduced after a 9 month administration of hypotensive doses of hydrochlorotiazide or perindopril (17). Thus, alterations in arterial wall structure and function occuring in hypertension seem to be reversible even at on old age. The reversibility seems to be dependent, however, on the blood pressure reduction per se, regardless how it is achieved.

Arterial Compliance

	Radial	Carotid	Aorta
CHF	↓	?	?
Hypercholesterolemia	↓	?	?
Hypothyroidism	↑	→	?
Diabetes	↓	↓	↓
Obesity	↑	?	?
Hypertension	↑	↓	?
ISH	↓	↓	?
Smoking	↓	↓	?
Training	↑	?	?
Menstrual Cycle *	↓	?	?

* luteinic phase

Figure 11.6: Radial, carotid and aortic compliance changes in several physiologic and pathologic conditions.

Arterial compliance in other conditions

Alterations of arterial compliance and, in particular, of radial artery compliance have been described in several other conditions (Figure 11.6). Some of these conditions deserve special attention because of their potential interaction with hypertension. This is the case for obesity, for example, which shows an increase in radial artery compliance before any blood pressure abnormality develops (18), raising the question of its mechanistic connection with the similar compliance alteration seen in hypertension. It is also the case for diabetes mellitus and hypercholesterolemia which are characterized, however, by an early marked reduction of arterial compliance (19, 20). Both conditions are more frequent in hypertension than in normotension which makes it important to determine whether and to what extent the resulting compliance values are affected. For the radial

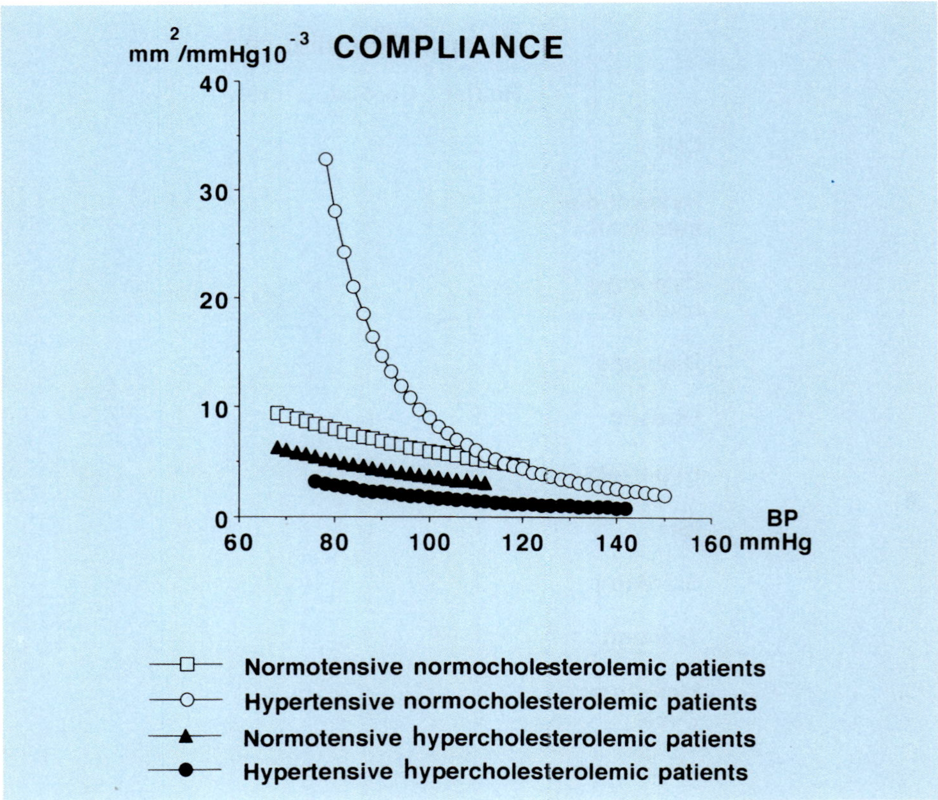

Figure 11.7: Cross-sectional compliance/blood pressure curves in one subject for each group of control, hypertensive normocholesterolemic, normotensive hypercholesterolemic, hypertensive hypercholesterolemic patients. Data from reference 21.

artery this has been investigated in subjects with normal blood pressure and serum cholesterol, high blood pressure and normal serum cholesterol, normal blood pressure and high serum cholesterol and high blood pressure and high serum cholesterol (Figure 11.7) (21). It is clear from the examples of Figure 11.7 that radial artery distensibility was decreased by hypercholesterolemia alone and increased by hypertension alone. The two conditions combined, however, reduced radial artery distensibility indicating that the effect of dyslipidemia on arterial function prevails over that of hypertension. This has pathophysiological implications because in hypertension an increased arterial compliance can be seen also as a mechanism absorbing and thus attenuating the traumatic effect of pressure on the vessel wall, thereby having an antiatherogenic effect. This is lost, however, whenever hypertension combines with dyslipidemia.

Finally, among the variety of structural and functional factors modulating radial artery compliance, sympathetic influences have been shown to play an important role, presumably by modulating contraction of vascular smooth muscle. This is documented by the observation that 1) infusion of phenylephrine in the brachial artery is accompanied by a reduction of radial artery compli-

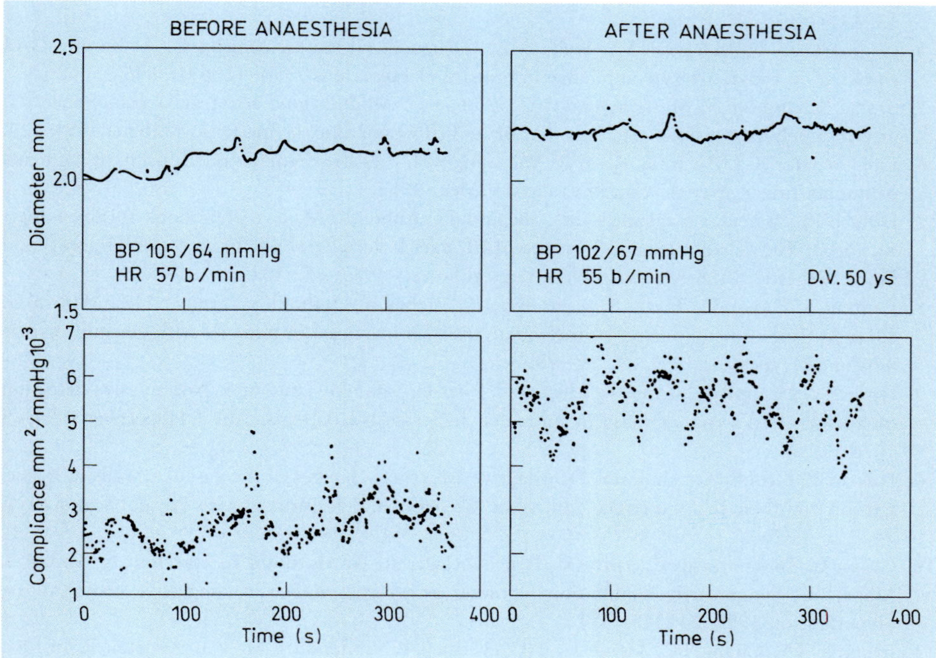

Figure 11.8: Beat-to-beat effect of the sympathetic blockade, by brachial plexus anaesthesia, on the diameter and the compliance of the radial artery. Data from reference 11.

ance, which is equally marked in normotensive and hypertensive subjects (Figure 11.3) (5); 2) stimuli acutely activating the sympathetic nervous system can also induce a marked reduction of radial artery compliance (4) and 3) removal of tonic sympathetic drive to the radial artery by anaesthesia of the brachial plexus, increases markedly compliance (Figure 11.8) (11). This may account at least in part for the evidence that in a condition characterized by sympathetic activation, such as congestive heart failure, radial artery compliance is decreased (22). It may also account for the marked improvement in compliance that is produced in congestive heart failure by ACE-inhibitor administration (23), given the ability of ACE-inhibition to remove the facilitating influence of angiotensin II on sympathetic vascular influences (24–27).

References

1. Mancia G, Failla M, Mangoni AA, Rivolta MR, Stella ML, Giannattasio C. Radial artery compliance in health and disease. High Blood Press 1994; 3: 217–221.
2. Tardy YJ, Meister JJ, Perret F, Brunner HR, Arditi M. Non invasive estimate of the mechanical properties of peripheral arteries from ultrasonic and photoplethysmographic measurements. Clin Phys Physiol Meas 1991; 3: 360–367.
3. Parati G, Casadei R, Groppelli A, Di Rienzo M, Mancia G. Comparison of finger and intra-arterial blood pressure monitoring at rest and during laboratory testing. Hypertension 1989; 13: 647–655.
4. Giannattasio C, Mangoni AA, Stella ML, Carugo S, Grassi G, Mancia G. Acute effects of smoking on radial artery compliance in humans. J Hypertens 1994; 12: 691–696.
5. Trazzi S, Omboni S, Mutti E, Parati G, Mancia G. Modulazione acuta della compliance (C) arteriosa nell'ipertensione arteriosa (IA) lieve. VIII Congr. Soc. It. Ipertens., Bologna 1991; 124.
6. Langewouters GJ, Zwart A, Busse R, Wesseling KH. Pressure diameter relationship of segments of human finger arteries. Clin Phys Physiol Meas 1986; 7: 43–45.
7. Dobrin PB. Vascular mechanics. In : Sheperd JT, Abboud FM, eds. Handbook of Physiology, section 2: The Cardiovascular System, vol III, part I: Peripheral Circulation and Organ Blood Flow. Bethesda, MD: American Physiological Society 1983; 65–102.
8. Laurent S, Hayoz D, Trazzi S, Boutouyrie P, Waeber B, Omboni S, Brunner HR, Mancia G, Safar M. Isobaric compliance of the radial artery is increased in patients with essential hypertension. J Hypertens 1993; 11: 89–98.
9. Girerd X, Mourad JJ, Copie X, Muolin C, Acar C, Safar M, Laurent S. Noninvasive detection of an increased vascular mass in untreated hypertensive patients. Am J Hypertens 1994; 7: 1076–1084.
10. Folkow B, Grimby G, Thulesius O. Adaptive structural changes of the vascular walls in hypertension and their relation to the control of the peripheral resistance. Acta Physiol Scand 1958; 44: 255–272.
11. Grassi G, Giannattasio C, Failla M, Pesenti A, Peretti G, Marinoni E, Fraschini N, Vailati S, Mancia G. Sympathetic modulation of radial artery compliance in congestive heart failure. Hypertension 1995; 26: 348–354.
12. Bruning TA, Chang PC, Hendriks MG, Vermeij P, Pfaffendorf M, van Zwieten P. In vivo characterization of muscarinic receptor subtypes that mediate vasodilatation in patients with essential hypertension. Hypertension 1995; 265(1): 70–77.
13. Reneman RS, Van Merode T, Hick PJJ, Muytjens AMM, Hoeks APG. Age related changes in carotid artery wall properties in men. Ultrasound Med Biol 1986; 12: 465–471.

14. Stella ML, Failla M, Mangoni AA, Carugo S, Scandola L, Grassi G, Giannattasio C, Mancia G. Differential effect of isolated systolic hypertension (ISH) and systo-diastolic hypertension (SDH) on compliance (C) of large and medium-size arteries. Seventh European Meeting on Hypertension, 184.
15. Mancia G, Ferrari AU, Giannattasio C, Trazzi S. Vascular effects of lacidipine: a review of animal and human data. J Hypertens 1993; 11(1): S39–S43.
16. Girerd X, Mourad JJ, Copie X, Moulin C, Acar C, Safar M, Laurent S. Noninvasive detection of an increased vascular mass in untreated hypertensive patients. Am J Hypertens 1994; 7: 1076–1084.
17. Girerd X, Giannattasio C, Moulin C, Safar M, Mancia G, Laurent S. Regression of radial artery wall hypertrophy and improvement of carotid artery compliance after long term antihypertensive treatment: the Pericles study. Seventh European Meeting on Hypertension, 69.
18. Managoni AA, Giannattasio C, Brunani A, Failla M, Colombo M, Bolla G, Cavagnini F, Grassi G, Mancia G. Radial artery compliance in young, obese, normotensive subjects. Hypertension 1995; 26: 984–988.
19. Giannattasio C, Gamba PL, Failla M, Mangoni AA, Carugo S, Scandola L, Maglia D, Piperno A, Paleari F, Mancia G. Early structural and functional alterations of radial and carotid arteries in IDDM. 16th International Society of Hypertension, Glasgow, in press.
20. Giannattasio C, Mangoni AA, Failla M, Carugo S, Stella ML, Stefanoni P, Grassi G, Vergani C, Mancia G. Impaired radial artery compliance in normotensive subjects with familial hypercholesterolemia. Atherosclerosis, 1996, in press.
21. Giannattasio C, Mangoni AA, Bombelli M, Stella ML, Carugo S, Grassi G, Mancia G. Effects of combined hypercholesterolemia and hypertension on arterial compliance. J Hypertens 1994; 12 (3): S217.
22. Giannattasio C, Failla M, Stella ML, Mangoni AA, Carugo S, Pozzi M, Grassi G, Mancia G. Alteration of radial artery compliance in patients with congestive heart failure. Am J Cardiol 1995; 76: 381–385.
23. Giannattasio C, Failla M, Stella ML, Mangoni AA, Turrini D, Carugo S, Pozzi M, Grassi G, Mancia G. Angiotensin converting enzyme inhibition and radial artery compliance in patients with congestive heart failure. Hypertension 1995; 26: 491–496.
24. Mancia G, Perondi R, Saino A, Tio R, Pomidossi G, Gregorini L, Zanchetti A. Hemodynamic effects of ACE inhibitors. Eur Heart J 1990; 11(D): 27–32.
25. Morganti A, Grassi G, Giannattasio C, Bolla GB, Turolo L, Saino A, Sala C, Mancia G, Zanchetti A. Effect of agiotensin converting enzyme inhibition on cardiovascular regulation during reflex sympathetic activation in sodium- replated patients with essential hypertension. J Hypertens 1989; 7: 825–835.
26. Giannattasio C, Cattaneo BM, Omboni S, Seravalle G, Bolla G, Turolo L, Morganti A, Grassi G, Zanchetti A, Mancia G. Sympathomoderating influence of benazepril in essential hypertension. J Hypertens 1992; 10: 373–378.
27. Perondi R, Saino A, Tio RA, Pomidossi G, Gregorini L, Alessio P, Morganti A, Zanchetti A, Mancia G. ACE-inhibition attenuates sympathetic coronary vasocostriction in patients with coronary artery diseases. Circulation 1992; 85: 2004–2013.

12 Arterial stiffness and extracellular matrix in ovariectomized female spontaneously hypertensive rats

Gerard M. London, Jean-Michel Courivaux, Michael Stimpel, Michel E. Safar

Introduction

Large-artery walls become thicker and stiffer in hypertension. Together with vascular smooth muscle cell hypertrophy, an increase in extracellular matrix involving principally elastin and collagen is also a major pathological and biochemical finding. Angiotensin converting enzyme (ACE) inhibitors seem to be more effective than other drugs in the regression or prevention of such arterial changes and might act independently of their antihypertensive action (1). Recent studies in SHR rats have demonstrated that ACE inhibitors prevent the development of aortic hypertrophy in a pressure-dependent manner whereas the development of collagen is prevented in a non-pressure dependent manner (2). However, these studies were performed exclusively in male spontaneously hypertensive rats (SHR). The finding might be different in males and females because the rate of extracellular matrix deposition appears to be higher in males than in females, and the administration of estrogen (beta-estradiol) to male hypertensive rats results in a decrease in connective tissue deposition and vascular hypertrophy (3,4). However, most studies have been performed in castrated male rats (5–10) and there are few data in females (11–13).

In a recent study, we compared male and female subjects with essential hypertension with regard to blood pressure levels and indices of arterial stiffening (14). In the studied population, pulse wave velocity (PWV) was measured non invasively in the aorta, the femoral and brachial arteries (Table 12.1). In non menopaused women, PWV was significantly lower than in age-matched men. In postmenopausal women, PWV was similar to that of age-matched men and this finding was associated with a significant age-related increase in wave reflections and systolic blood pressure. From these data, it was suggested that, in postmenopausal women, the similar value of PWV as that of age-matched men was due to the loss of estrogen's protective effect. In addition, because PWV increased markedly after menopause, the resulting increase in aortic wave reflections could be responsible for the steeper age-related increase in systolic blood pressure observed in postmenopausal women.

Table 12.1: Clinical and arterial parameters in non menopaused and postmenopausal women and age-matched men (14).

	Non menopaused women (n = 44)	Men (n = 44)	Post-menopausal women (n = 24)	Men (n = 40)
Age (years)	34.7 ± 8.8	32.0 ± 9.5	64.8 ± 10.7	64.6 ± 15.2
Weight (kg)	57.3 ± 9.1	75.2 ± 9.6***	60.1 ± 8.4	74.5 ± 13.5***
Height (cm)	161.8 ± 8.2	177.5 ± 7.0***	154.3 ± 7.0	170.8 ± 8.1***
Systolic BP (mmHg)	125.4 ± 14.6	134.4 ± 18.2**	145.3 ± 22.0	144.4 ± 21.4
Diastolic BP (mmHg)	75.6 ± 10.8	81.3 ± 12.3*	80.7 ± 11.7	82.8 ± 11.4
Aortic PWV (cm/sec)	752 ± 111	802 ± 136*	1031 ± 159	1032 ± 201
Femoral PWV (cm/sec)	957 ± 98	1049 ± 130***	1113 ± 136	1104 ± 131
Brachial PWV (cm/sec)	982 ± 119	1055 ± 168*	1085 ± 139	1135 ± 149

Mean values ± SD.
Abbreviations are: BP, blood pressure; PWV, pulse wave velocity; +P < 0.05; **P < 0.01; ***P < 0.001 (men versus women).

Taken together, the observed findings in humans and rats indicate that: (i) the increased arterial stiffness in both sexes seems to be strongly related to the extent of connective tissue within the arterial wall, (ii) the development of arterial stiffness differs significantly in men and women, with a greater age-related increase in stiffness in postmenopausal women, (iii) the increase in stiffness in postmenopausal women is possibly due to the loss of estrogen's protection with a resulting change in extracellular matrix of the arterial wall. Finally, the question is raised to know whether the extracellular matrix of arterial vessels in females is modulated, independently of blood pressure changes, by estrogen therapy, converting enzyme inhibition, or a combination of both factors.

The purpose of the present study was to show that: (i) the development of the collagen and elastin contents of the arterial wall is different in males and females, suggesting a specific contribution of female sexual hormones, and (ii) in female SHRs studied in the presence or absence of ovarian glands, ACE inhibition is able to prevent the collagen and/or elastin accumulation of the arterial wall independently of blood pressure changes.

Methods

Animals

Four week-old SHRs (Iffa-Credo, L'Abresle, France) were randomly allocated into 6 groups (n = 8 per group). Two groups of male SHRs were treated by placebo or by the ACE inhibitor moexipril, respectively, the latter given at an anthypertensively effective dose (for dosages: see below). Two other groups were composed of female SHRs divided into the same subgroups according to the 2 varieties of treatment. Finally, the last two groups were composed of ovariectomized SHRs divided into the same subgroups according to treatment. Ovariectomy was performed previous to the investigation. All rats were housed 4–5 per cage in an animal room (temperature, 20° to 22 °C; humidity, 55% to 65%; 12-hour light/dark cycle), fed a standard diet (0.1 mEq/g Na^+ and 0.205 mEq/g K^+), and had free access to tap water.

Dose treatments

Vehicle ("placebo") or oral moexipril at 10 mg/kg/day were administered for 16 weeks. The volumes administered were similar in the various groups and did not exceed 0.5 ml/100 g body wt per day. The dose of moexipril used in this study had been indentified in an earlier dose-response study in SHRs as being the most balanced in terms of good antihypertensive efficacy on the one hand and absence of toxicity on the other (2).

Study design

During the treatment period, systolic blood pressure (SBP) was measured noninvasively by a tail-cuff method at 8, 12 and 16 weeks of age. Five consecutive measurements were performed at each control, and the mean of these values was considered. When the difference was higher than 15 mmHg, the measurements were started again.

At the end of the treatment period, the animals were sacrificed and the thoracic aortas were used for the evaluation of histomorphological parameters. The procedures followed in this study are in accordance with institutional guidelines of animal experiments.

Morphological study

Histomorphometric parameters of the thoracic aorta were measured at 20 weeks of age according to the following procedure. The animals were anaesthetized with pentobarbital, and then after median thoracotomy, they were exsanguinated by the mean of a catheter placed in the right auricle whereas saline was injected by the femoral catheter. When the liquid coming from the auricle was clear, the circulatory tract was rinsed with a 4% formaldehyde buffered solution. The animals died within seconds after starting formaldehyde infusion. After 1 or 2 minutes, a clamp was positioned on the auricle and the fixation liquid was infused for 3 hours at a pressure equal to the mean blood pressure

(MBP) of each animal. At the end of the perfusion, the thoracic aorta was dissected and preserved in a 4% formaldehyde solution until the histological study was performed.

The different structures of the aortic media were studied in a segment of thoracic aorta longitudinally embedded in paraffin. Three successive sagittal sections of 5 μm thickness were treated by specific staining to obtain a monochromatic color associated with the various structures studied in the aortic media. Sirius red was used for collagen staining, orcein for elastin, and hematoxylin after periodic acid oxidation for nucleus staining. Morphometric analysis was performed with a specialized automated image processor (NS 1500, Nachet-Vision, Paris, France). This processor is based upon morphological mathematics principles and is software controlled. Different algorithms were developed to analyze each of the three structures shown by the staining in each of the three successive sections. For image processing, the image is sent to the processor via a video camera and can be viewed on the TV monitor. The control of luminosity was automatically adjusted by the software in order to obtain similar contrasts, taking into account the total luminosity transmitted by the video camera. This analogue image is then digitized as follows: each elementary point (pixel) is automatically compared with a threshold; if the grey level of pixel exceeds this threshold, the pixel is given numeric value 1, otherwise it is given the numeric value 0. Threshold parameters are the size of such pixel groups and their local contrast (top-hat transformation). The threshold was determined using the top-hat transformation algorithm so as to minimize variations in nuclear staining and background.

For data processing, this binary image is then processed to: 1) eliminate background and artifacts, 2) delineate the zones of interest and the reference zone, 3) extract and measure the parameters form the various zones of interest.

The first algorithm permitted to analyze the mean media thickness by measurements of the distance between the internal and external elastic lamina (70 measurements in each section). Medial elastin network was analyzed in terms of relative area and mean thickness of elastin lamella and lamina; the measurements and calculations were made in 10 fields in each section. The second algorithm analyzed the collagen matrix by measurement of relative area density of collagen fibers in 20 contiguous fields in each Sirius red stained section. Elastin and collagen densities were defined as the ratio of the surface stained by orcein or Sirius red, respectively, to the surface of the studied field. Elastin and collagen contents were calculated as the density multiplied by media-thickness. The third algorithm counted the number of nuclei within 20 fields of 10,000 μm^2/area of measurement in each section and measured the mean area of each nucleus. A two-step procedure (conditional opening, then conditional closing) leads to the elimination of all particles under a predetermined size. The final result is retention of the image of the nuclei, without any holes or deformations due to the structuring element (hexagon). The image processor automatically eliminates border line nuclei, before making the measurement of the number of nuclei/unit of surface. Repetitive measurements were performed, pooled and averaged for the three algorithms in the corresponding stained sections of the aortic wall media of each animal. Morphological analysis were performed twice in a blind fashion by two independent persons.

Statistical analysis

Results were expressed as mean ± SD. Using a statistical logiciel, data were analyzed with a two-way analysis of variance (treatment and gender effects). When F was less than 0.05, a LSD test was performed for intergroup comparison. P values ≤ 0.05 were considered as significant.

Result

Figure 12.1 summarizes the changes in body weight. Body weight during the follow-up was constantly lower in females than in males, particularly in non-ovariectomized females, but there was no drug effect on the body weight changes during the follow-up.

Figure 12.2 indicates that, in untreated animals, hypertension was fully developed in SHRs either males or females (with or without ovariectomy). Systolic blood pressure was constantly and significantly higher in males than in females ($P < 0.001$), with insignificant differences between females according to the presence or absence of ovariectomy. Moexipril caused a significant antihypertensive effect either in males or females, with or without ovariectomy.

Table 12.2 summarizes the histomorphometric findings on aortic thickness, collagen and elastin contents and nuclei size.

Arterial thickness was constantly lower in females than in males ($P < 0.003$). In treated SHRs, the reduction in thickness was more pronounced in ovariectomized females by comparison with non-ovariectomized females. Treatment reduced significantly arterial thickness (0.0000).

Elastin content was significantly reduced by treatment ($P = 0.0000$). Elastin content was significantly more reduced in ovariectomized females, than in males and in non ovariectomized females ($P = 0.001$). This finding was not influenced by treatment.

There was no sex effect for collagen content. Collagen content was significantly reduced by treatment, particularly for males ($P = 0.004$). For nuclei size, there was a significant sex-effect, but not a drug-effect.

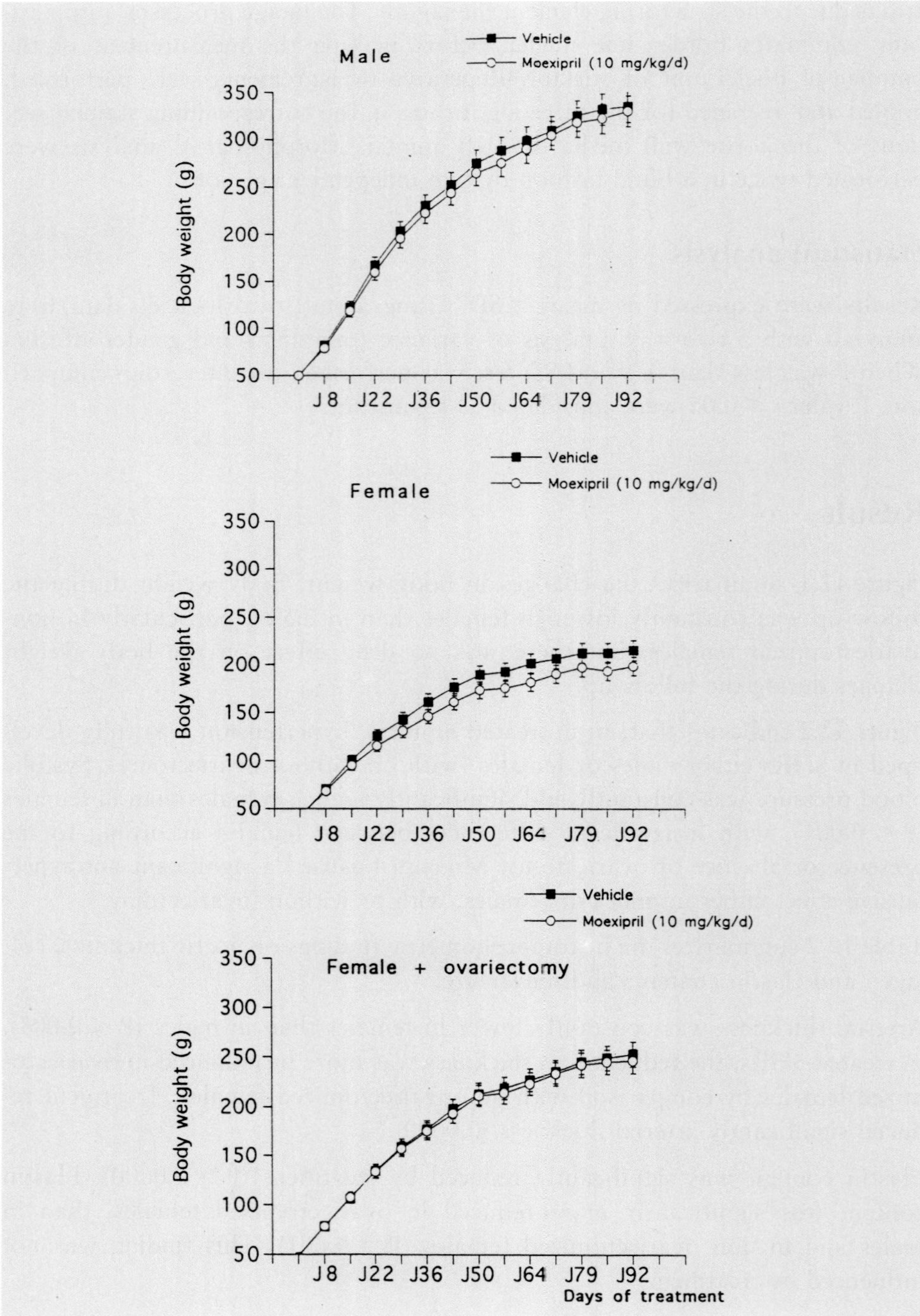

Figure 12.1: Follow-up of male and female SHRs: changes in body weight.

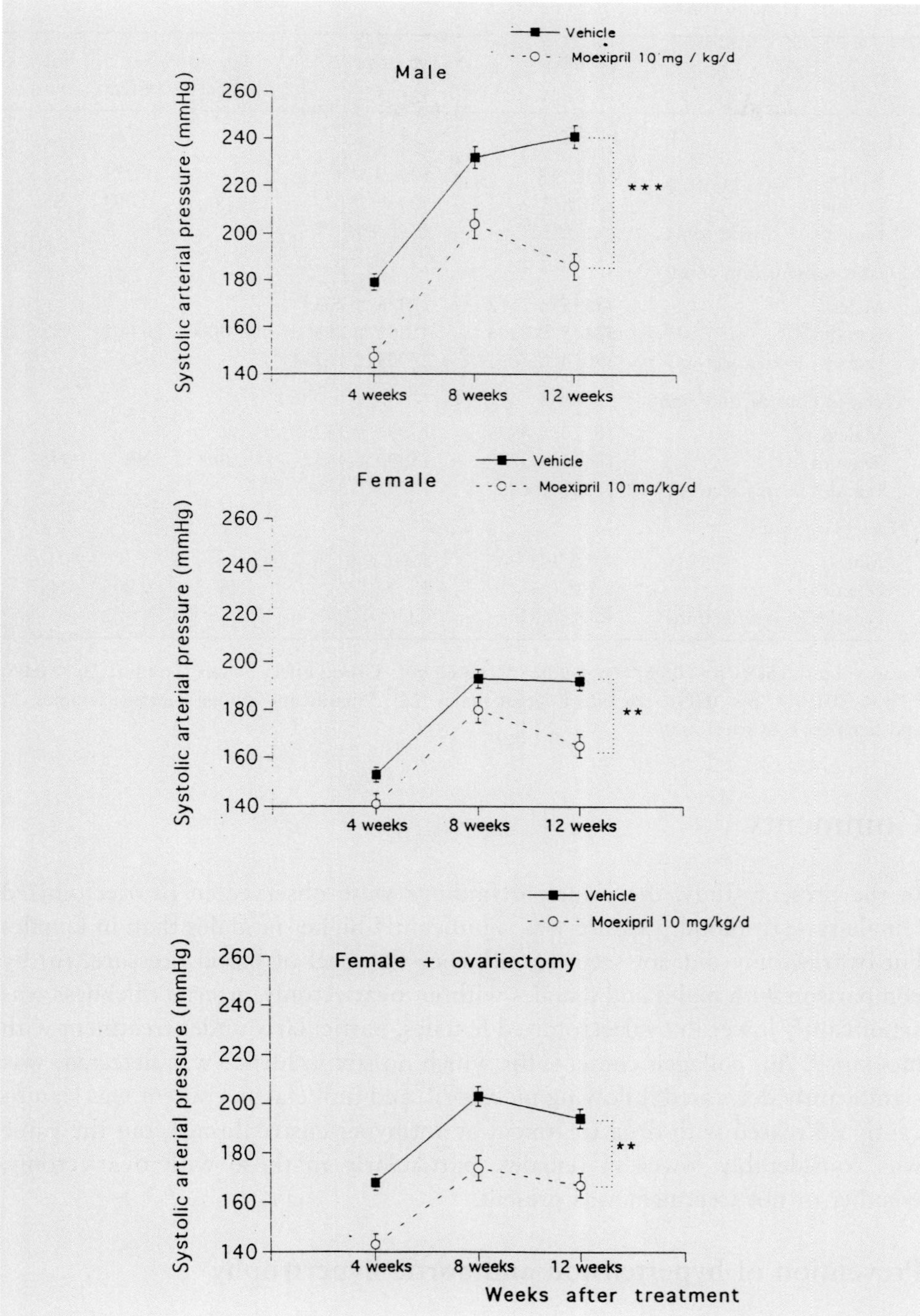

Figure 12.2: Follow-up of male and female SHRs: changes in systolic blood pressure (**$p < 0.01$; ***$P < 0.001$).

Table 12.2: Histomorphometric parameters.

	Placebo	Moexipril	Group effect	Sex effect	Interaction
Thickness (μm)					
Males	131± 18	109 ± 5**			
Females	120 ± 7+	105 ± 7**	0.0000	0.003	NS
Females + ovariectomy	111 ± 5++	93 ± 1***+•			
Elastin content (μm^2/mm)					
Males	48595 ± 7572	38076 ± 2663*			
Females	52445 ± 6294	41861 ± 10808*	0.0000	0.001	NS
Females + ovariectomy	39054 ± 7631+•	27003 ± 1623**•			
Collagen content (μm^2/mm)					
Males	20120 ± 4879	15984 ± 2225**			
Females	18621 ± 3749	15970 ± 1152	0.004	NS	NS
Females + ovariectomy	17621 ± 642	13793 ± 1406*			
Nuclei size (μm^2)					
Males	4.9 ± 0.5	5.4 ± 0.6			
Females	5.5 ± 0.6	5.6 ± 0.3	NS	0.008	NS
Females + ovariectomy	4.3 ± 0.83	4.6 ± 0.7			

Mean values ± SD; $^{*}p < 0.05$; $^{**}p < 0.01$; $^{***}p < 0.001$. Group effect versus Group I; $^{+}p < 0.05$; $^{++}p < 0.01$; $^{+++}p < 0.001$. Sex effect versus males (M); •Significant change between females (F) and females + ovariectomy.

Comments

In the present study, the principal findings were observed in ovariectomized female rats: (i) blood pressure was significantly higher in males than in females but ovariectomy did not seem to influence the level of blood pressure, (ii) by comparison with males and females without ovariectomy, arterial thickness was significantly lower in ovariectomized females, particularly under treatment with moexipril, (iii) collagen content, for which no sex influence was detected, was significantly decreased following moexipril, and (iiii) elastin content was significantly decreased with drug treatment at antihypertensive dosage, but the value was considerably lower in females, particularly in those with ovariectomy, whether or not treatment was present.

Prevention of hypertension and aortic hypertrophy

Our results show that moexipril was able to prevent the development of genetic hypertension in male, female, and ovariectomized female SHRs. In addition, placebo treated hypertensive animals developed a significant aortic medial hypertrophy, with values comparable to those observed by others in SHRs of the same age (2). Hypertrophy of the thoracic aorta was prevented by moexipril. We have previously reported that in parallel with the blood pressure reduction, converting enzyme inhibitors and hydralazine displayed similar effects on aortic hypertrophy in male SHRs (2). These findings strongly suggested that, in the present genetic model of hypertension, prevention of aortic hypertrophy may depend principally on the effect of drugs on blood pressure level. However, the present study also suggests a gender influence on aortic medial hypertrophy, since arterial thickness was significantly lower in ovariectomized than in non-ovariectomized female SHRs at the same level of blood pressure in both groups, treated (moexipril) or untreated (vehicle).

Thus, besides blood pressure reduction, sex hormones played a significant effect on aortic structures, which was independant of treatment.

Prevention of aortic collagen accumulation

In a previous work (2), we showed in male SHRs that the converting enzyme inhibitor quinapril was able to prevent aortic collagen accumulation, under the same conditions as in the present work. The effect was shown to be pressure independent, since the same degree of prevention was observed with a low or a high dose of quinapril. In the present work, the effect on collagen accumulation could be also extended to females. In female SHRs with or without ovariectomy, the prevention of collagen accumulation was less pronounced as compared to males, but here, the relatively small number of animals might be responsible for a loss of statistical power. Interestingly, there was no sex effect for aortic collagen accumulation, i. e. sexual hormones did not seem to have a major influence on collagen metabolism within the limits of the present experiment.

Prevention of aortic elastin

ACE inhibitors have been shown to decrease elastin content in SHRs but the finding seemed to be of lesser degree than that for collagen. On the other hand, results of the literature were restricted to males (3–10). The present work clearly shows that there is a distinct sex influence for elastin content in SHRs. Firstly, whereas, in placebo-treated animals, elastin content was quite similar in males and females without ovariectomy, a significant decrease was observed in placebo-treated females with ovariectomy. Secondly, this decrease was even more pronounced in ovariectomized females treated by converting enzyme inhibition. In ovariectomized females, it seems that the distinct reduction in elastin content following moexipril was neither the simple consequence of blood pressure reduction, nor was it due to the exclusive role of converting enzyme inhibition. It seems rather that a specific interaction was present between converting enzyme inhibition and sex hormones. In the literature, one study on cultured chick embryonic arterial smooth muscle cells has shown that angiotensin II inhibited elastin synthesis through the interaction of its receptor and the modulation of intracellular calcium (15).

Whatever the mechanisms involved, it appears that the decrease in elastin content in ovariectomized female SHRs might contribute per se to increase the arterial rigidity. Some findings in the literature strengthen this interpretation. Firstly, the turn-over and accumulation of collagen and elastin in aorta has been previously determined in ovariectomized female WKY rats (11, 12). The conclusion was that estradiol increased the degradation of both collagen and elastin in rat aorta, resulting in a lower total accumulation of both these fibers but with a higher proportion of the elastic fibers, thus decreasing the stiffness of the vessel wall. Secondly, studies of the passive mechanical properties of the carotid artery in male normotensive castrated rats have indicated that estradiol decreases the stiffness of arteries (9). Finally, it is noteworthy that several recent studies have assessed the presence of estrogen receptors within the arterial wall (16, 17). Thus, such findings agree with our clinical observation that arterial rigidity increases markedly in postmenopausal women. However, several important problems yet remain to be resolved. These problems are: (i) the exact mechanism of the estrogen induced changes in arterial stiffness in postmenopausal women and in ovariectomized female rats, (ii) the possible interactions of the estrogen induced arterial changes with aging and hypertension, and (iii) the relationship between sex hormones and converting enzyme inhibition, specifically as far as arterial elastin and collagen are concerned.

Acknowledgments

The study was performed with a grant from the Assistance Publique de Paris, the Institut National de la Santé et de la Recherche Médicale (INSERM, U 337), the Association Claude Bernard and the Ministère de la Recherche, Paris. We thank Mrs. Annette Seban for her excellent assistance

References

1. Safar ME, Levy BI. The response of large arteries to antihypertensive therapy: I basic concepts. In O'Rourke M, Safar ME, Dzau VJ (eds.): Arterial vasodilation, mechanisms and therapy. Edward Arnold pub, London, 1993: 149–156.
2. Albaladejo P, Bouaziz H, Duriez M, Gohlke P, Levy B, Safar M, Benetos A. Angiotensin converting enzyme inhibition prevents the increase in aortic collagen in rats. Hypertension 1994; 23: 74–82.
3. Wolinsky H. Comparative effects of castration and anti-androgen treatment on the response of the aortic wall to hypertension. Circ Res 1973; 33: 183–181.
4. Wolinsky H. Response of the rat aortic media to hypertension: morphological and clinical studies. Circ Res 1970; 26: 507–512.

5. Fischer GM, Swain ML. Effect of sex hormones on blood pressure and vascular connective tissue in castrated and noncastrated male rats. Am J Physiol 1977; 232: H617–H621.
6. Fischer GM, Cherian K, Swain ML. Increased synthesis of aortic collagen and elastin in experimental atherosclerosis. Inhibition by contraceptive steroids. Atherosclerosis 1981; 39: 463–467.
7. Fischer GM, Swain ML. In vivo effects of sex hormones on aortic elastin and collagen dynamics in castrated and intact male rats. Endocrinology 1978; 10: 92–97.
8. Wolinsky H, Goldfischer S, Schiller B, Kasak LE. Modification of the effects of hypertension on lysosomes and connective tissue in the rat aorta Circ Res 1973; 34: 233–241.
9. Cox RH, Fischer GM. Effects of sex hormones on the passive mechanical properties of rat carotid artery. Blood Vessels 1978; 15: 266–276.
10. Wolinsky H. Effects of estrogen and progestogen treatment on the response of the aorta of male rats to hypertension. Morphological and chemical studies. Circ Res 1972; 30: 341–349.
11. Fischer GM, Swain ML. Influence of contraceptive and other sex steroids on aortic collagen and elastin. Exp Mol Pathol 1980; 33: 15–24.
12. Fischer GM. In vivo effects of estradiol on collagen and elastin dynamics in rat aorta. Endocrinology 1972; 91: 1227–1232.
13. Wolinsky H. Effects of estrogen treatment on the oophorectomized female rat aorta. P.E.S E.B.M. 1973; 144: 864–867.
14. London G, Guérin A, Pannier B, Marchais S, Stimpel M. Influence of sex on arterial hemodynamics and blood pressure. Role of body height. Hypertension 1995; 16: 514–519.
15. Tokimitsu I, Kato H, Wachi H, Tajima S. Elastin synthesis is inhibited by angiotensin II but not by platelet-derived growth factor in arterial smooth muscle cells. Biochem Biophys Acta – Protein Structure and Molecular enzymology 1994; 1207: 68–73.
16. Kangar KF ; Vyas S, Whitehead M, Crook D, Meire H, Campbell S. Pulsatility index in internal carotid artery in relation to transdermal oestradiol and time since menopause. Lancet 1991; 338: 839–842.
17. Mendelsohn ME, Karas RH. Estrogen and the blood vessel wall. Curr Opin Cardiol 1994; 9: 619–626.